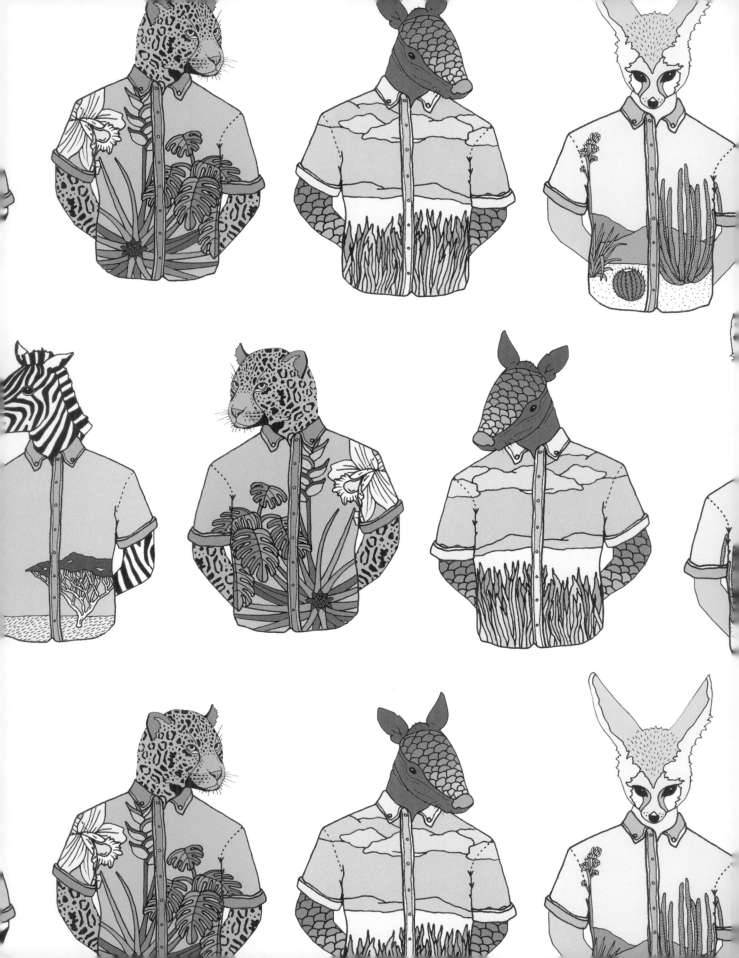

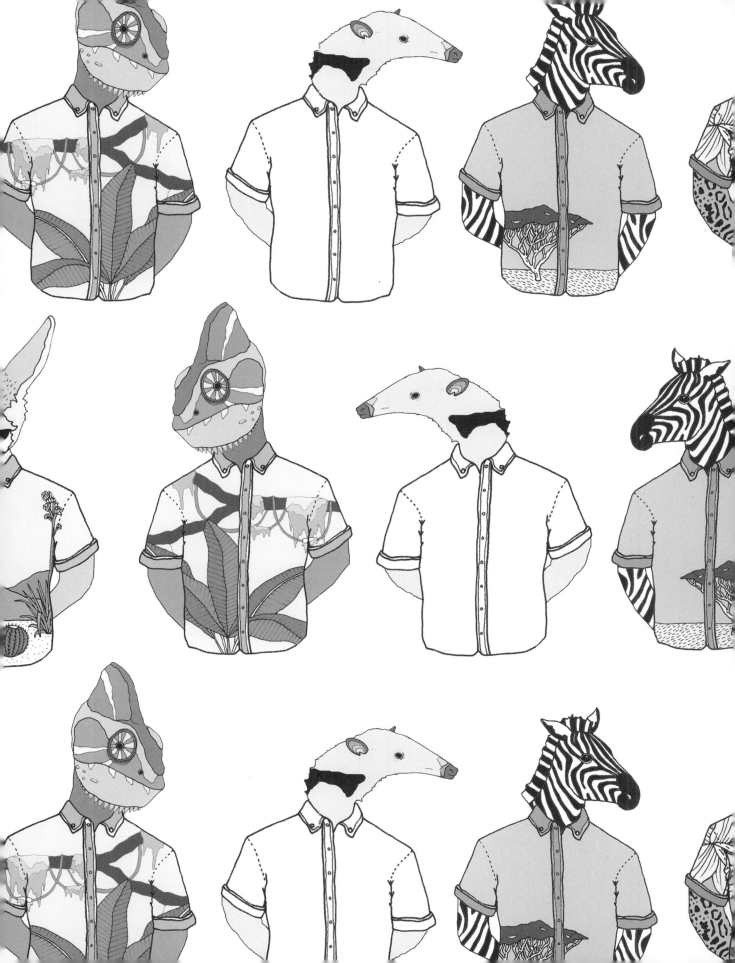

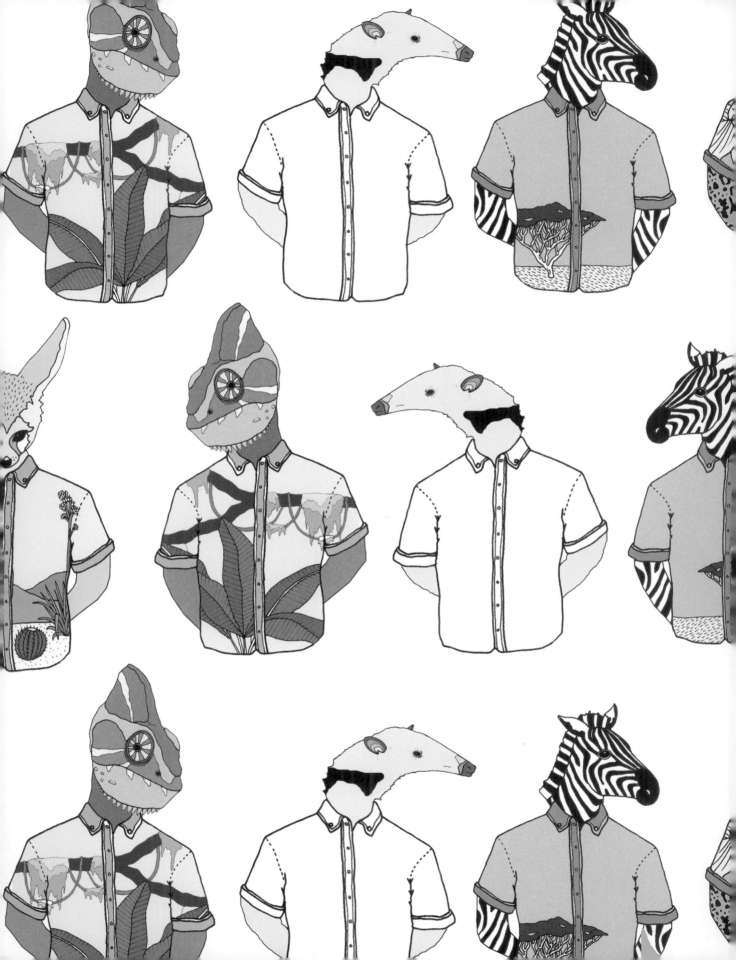

Seeing Gender

There are sections of this book that may be hard to read. Many of these might be highly personal, so I am unable to identify everything in the book that might be upsetting, but I can point out in particular pages 120-125 as well as 132 that cover more intense subjects. Please use your own discretion while reading this book, and I encourage you to skip what feels like too much.

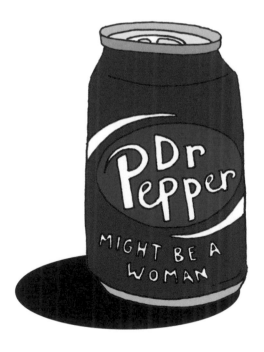

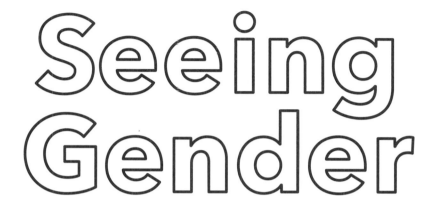

Seeing Gender

An Illustrated Guide to
Identity and Expression

By Iris Gottlieb

Foreword by National Book Award Winner
and Stonewall Book Award Honoree Kacen Callender

CHRONICLE BOOKS

SAN FRANCISCO

To all of us who are figuring it out (and Bunny the dog).

First Chronicle Books LLC paperback edition, published in 2022.

Originally published in hardcover in 2019 by Chronicle Books LLC.

Text and Illustration copyright © 2019, 2022 by Iris Gottlieb.
Foreword copyright © 2022 by Kacen Callender.

Library of Congress Cataloging-in-Publication Data available.

ISBN 978-1-7972-1197-8

Manufactured in China.

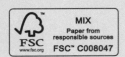

Original Book Design by Kelly Abeln and Michael Morris.
Paperback Design by Jay Marvel.

10 9 8 7 6 5 4 3 2

Chronicle books and gifts are available at special quantity discounts to corporations, professional associations, literacy programs, and other organizations. For details and discount information, please contact our premiums department at corporatesales@chroniclebooks.com or at 1-800-759-0190.

Chronicle Books LLC
680 Second Street
San Francisco, California 94107

Chronicle Books—we see things differently. Become part of our community at www.chroniclebooks.com/teen.

Contents

Foreword

By Kacen Callender

When I was a teenager, I *hated* gender roles—hated when people had expectations of me, or had preconceived ideas of who I was based on the three oversimplified words a doctor said at the time of my birth: "It's a girl!" (At least, I'm assuming the doctor said that when I was born. I don't know for sure. I was just a baby.)

The only problem was, as a teen, I didn't have the tools to explain why I hated gender roles so much. I didn't have the facts and data I definitely could have used in my many debates and arguments against toxic masculinity. I hadn't even begun to realize that I longed for people to look at me and not automatically assume my gender, or who I was because of my gender—hadn't known then that these thoughts and feelings were the beginnings of my own exploration into my gender identity as a non-binary demiboy.

It's a massive understatement to say I would've loved to have a gift like *Seeing Gender* back then—not only to give me the language and tools to empower myself and help me understand my identity, but to understand gender in a way that isn't taught enough.

This collection of thoughts, facts, illustrations, emotions, and personal story weaves together a tapestry that feels like an expression of gender itself: amorphous, ever-changing, bodies dancing in celebration of themselves, souls longing for the freedom from the boxes we're often forced into.

A book like *Seeing Gender* is a key to open the box, the door, to exploration—to seeing our true selves through free expression of identity. Isn't that really what every human wants in the end? So many of us long for the freedom to be our true selves, regardless of expectation from others, and especially when those expectations are created because of the three words a doctor says at our birth.

Seeing Gender is a necessary combination of historical, eye-opening fact, and human feeling and experience. We're gifted tools to break down the boxes that attempt to limit who we are, sharing with us history that explains many of the lies that created the foundation of the cage so many of us are trapped in; modern-day facts that are a blueprint of the cage so that we can dismantle it; fun facts that add sparks of joy along the way, a reminder that even as we sometimes struggle to free ourselves from these cages, our explorations and expressions of our identities can be fun and beautiful.

My hope for any reader who picks up this book is that they feel the same deep empathy I began to feel for myself as I read, as a trans masculine person who still feels the layers of boxes of expectation, the "rules" of gender, and wishes we could all break free and do exactly as we please, be who we truly are without fear. One of my favorite passages described how many different trans and non-binary identities have been seen as healers throughout history. It's fitting that the author has created a book, then, that is so healing—not only for transgender and non-binary readers, but for cisgender readers, too, to help us understand how our societies came to our current understanding of gender, and to shine a light on a path to freedom for us all.

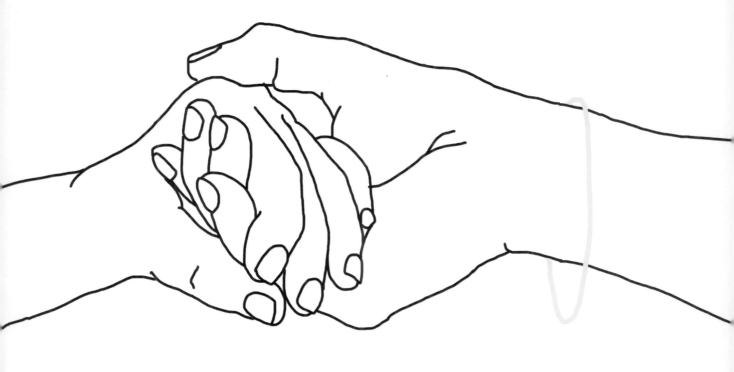

Introduction

Gender is complex, as are all facets of humanity. Humans invented gender, so we should do our best to understand it.

I am not a scholar of gender studies, but I have a gender and a body, as do you. Every person who might look at this page has the experience of inhabiting a body in a gendered world. I felt compelled to write this book during my own experience of shifting from being completely apathetic about my own gender to being knee-deep in wading through its ongoing transformation. Drawing helped me to process my bodily experiences and connect with people around the world through social media about this intense y personal and sensitive topic. Because so much of gender is visually oriented, it seems fitting to convey these abstract and amorphous concepts through the universal language of illustration.

This book is many things:

- An accessible entry point to understanding the vast complexities and histories of gender expression.

- A self-education tool that will allow for non-judgmental exploration of your own gender, increased empathy and understanding of others' experiences, and an invitation to consider the intricacies of intersectionality.

- A look into how coexisting identities (race, class, gender, sexuality, mental health) relate to gender within larger social systems.

- The story of my gender and how it changed over time, as well as stories from a wide range of people about their gender identities, difficulties, thoughts, and experiences—punctuated by some really good outfits.

- A hand of reassurance in the big, dark, scary abyss of finding oneself in the world. It cannot be underestimated, the power of seeing yourself in other people and feeling less alone in alienating experiences. For the queer, transgender, asexual, uncertain, self-conscious people looking at this, you are not alone!

In writing this book, I want to help build empathy and understanding among those who are not familiar with people who fall outside the lines of binary genders by telling personal stories, giving facts and history, and praising revolutionaries. I'll also be revealing the difficulties of embodying these genders, because we cannot only feel the joy of something in its most positive moments unless we also feel the sadness and hardship in its darkest.

The purpose of this book is to synthesize information about a huge and complex topic into an accessible and beautiful format that is explained from a non-academic, intersectional perspective. Some of the information is personal and is meant to be interpreted as such. All experiences of living in one's body are unique and personal. This book makes every effort to include as many perspectives as possible, with the knowledge that some voices will be missed or inaccurately portrayed. To anyone who reads this and does not feel represented, I am very sorry and hope to learn more from this experience.

Hello

About Me

NAME: Iris Gottlieb

AGE: 30

PRONOUN: She/her (for now)

FROM: Durham, North Carolina

RACE: White

GENDER IDENTITY: Boy (for now)

FAVORITE ICE CREAM: Cookies 'n' cream

PROFESSION: Illustrator, writer, scientist, grump, animator

FAVORITE OBJECT: My collection of four thousand found shark teeth

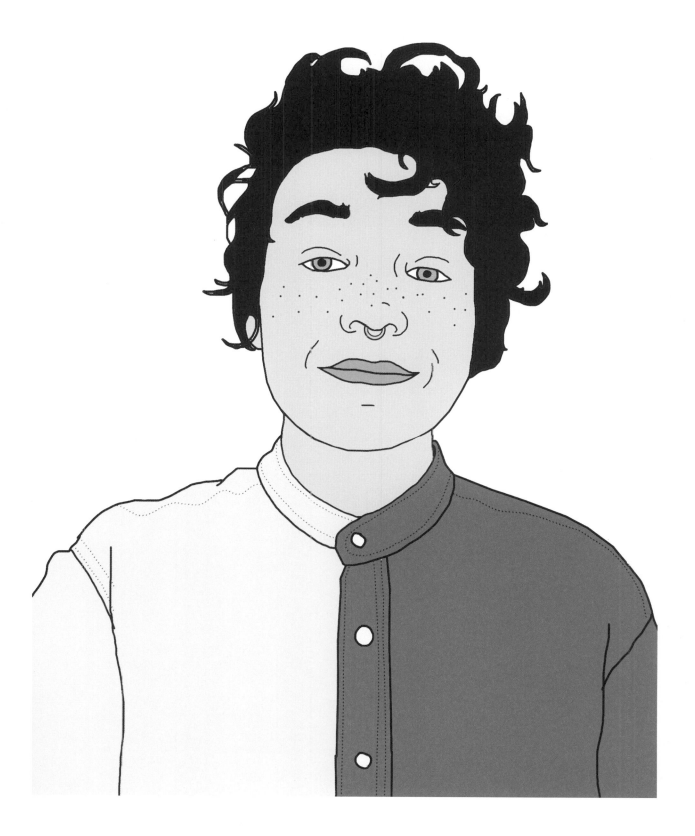

A Good Place to Start

Gender Is a Social Construct

Humans invented gender.

We also invented written language, math, religion, race, and measured time. These concepts are relevant and important, but exist only within the scope of humanity. We get to break the rules of gender because they aren't real and are often harmful. By not playing by gender rules, we move away from gender being necessary and toward everyone living life unabashedly and unafraid in the body they want, loving whom they want, and dressing how they want.

We've gotta learn to undo our own creation . . . or at least try.

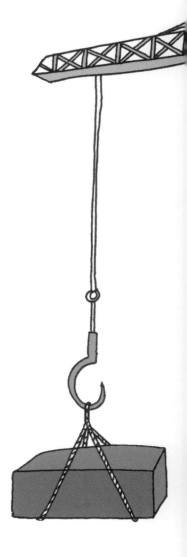

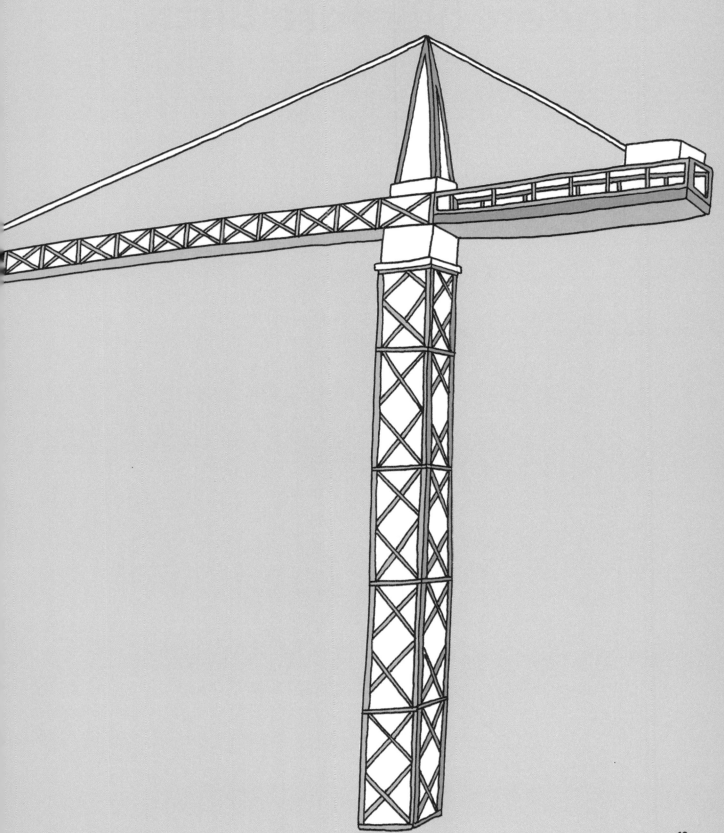

Gendered Before Birth

Gender is the first piece of data we gather about a person, the first inquiry from the outside world of who we will turn out to be. This inquiry begins before we are even born and continues thereafter.

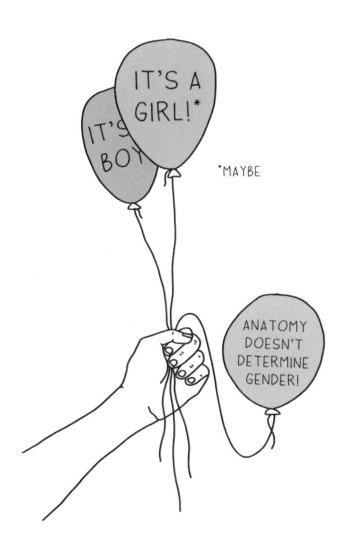

Temperature-Dependent Sex Determination:

A Note About Baby Sea Turtles

In most species, sex is determined during fertilization. However, the sex of baby sea turtles (and a handful of other reptiles) is determined by the temperature of the area in which their fertilized eggs are laid. If the surrounding sand is consistently cooler than approximately 82 degrees Fahrenheit, there will be mostly males; if it's above approximately 88 degrees Fahrenheit, there will be mostly females. If the temperature fluctuates, it will be a mixed group.

Climate change is causing warmer sand temperatures and therefore a disproportionate ratio of females to males, making reproduction more difficult.

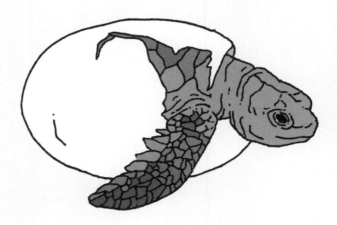

Introduction to Some Terminology

Note: *This is not meant to be an exhaustive list of definitions, but a guide to start you on your way.*

Agender: Not identifying with any gender.

Aromantic: Experiencing little or no romantic interest in others (this is a spectrum).

Asexual: Experiencing little or no sexual attraction to others, or low or absent desire for sexual activity. Not all asexual people are aromantic (one is a sexuality, one is a romantic attraction). Asexuality is different from celibacy! Celibacy is an intentional choice to abstain from sex; asexuality is not.

Assigned gender at birth (AGAB): The gender identity assigned to an individual at birth based on their biological sex characteristics. It may or may not align with a person's true gender identity. Some trans and non-binary people find it helpful to use the terms AMAB (assigned male at birth) or AFAB (assigned female at birth) to describe their experiences, while others may find such labels counterproductive. It's ultimately a matter of personal preference.

Biological sex: The physical characteristics of reproductive organs, secondary sexual characteristics, chromosomes, and hormones. This is not binary.

Bisexual: Attracted to both men and women; also sometimes defined as attraction to more than one gender, or attraction to the same gender and other genders.

Butch: Someone who mentally, emotionally, and/or physically identifies as masculine. Often applies to queer women.

(Cis)gender: Someone whose gender identity and sex assigned at birth are the same.

Demi-: A prefix used to indicate partial association with an identity. For example, a *demisexual* only experiences *some* sexual attraction (often based on emotional connections), and a *demigirl* may identify *mostly* as a girl, but not entirely.

Drag queen/king: A man who dresses in women's clothes, or a woman who dresses in men's clothes, usually for entertainment. Being a drag queen/king does not indicate someone's sexual orientation or gender identity, though it is usually associated with queer/gay communities.

Femme: Someone who mentally, emotionally, and/or physically identifies as feminine.

Gender binary: The idea that there are only two genders: male and female.

Gender dysphoria: The feeling that one's body and one's gender identity are misaligned.

Gender expression: How one displays their gender through dress, social behavior, and/or demeanor.

Gender fluid: Someone whose gender varies and is expressed dynamically.

Gender identity: The internal feeling of one's gender. This can be different from gender expression and gender assigned at birth. Some common identities are woman, man, transgender, genderqueer, agender.

Genderqueer: Someone who does not identify with the gender binary. This is often used as an umbrella term that includes gender fluid, agender, gender non-conforming, etc.

Heteronormativity: Though this term originally described the assumption that all people are heterosexual, the definition has expanded to encompass assumptions about gender. Heteronormativity manifests institutionally (gendered bathrooms or not including gender-neutral options on forms) and socially (asking a male-presenting person, "Do you have a girlfriend?" or having a bachelorette party with dick-shaped candy).

Heterosexual: Someone who is exclusively physically attracted to people of the "opposite sex" within the gender binary/heteronormativity.

Homosexual: Someone who is attracted physically and emotionally to people of the same sex. Note: This word is not used much anymore, as queer, gay, and LGBTQIA+ are generally accepted in the vernacular now.

Intersex (formerly hermaphrodite): "A general term used for a variety of conditions in which a person is born with a reproductive or sexual anatomy that doesn't seem to fit the typical definitions of female or male."—Intersex Society of North America

Non-binary: Someone who does not identify with the gender binary. As the National Center for Transgender Equality says, "People . . . use many different terms to describe themselves, with non-binary being one of the most common. Other terms include genderqueer, agender, bigender, and more. None of these terms mean exactly the same thing—but all speak to an experience of gender."

Pronouns: The pronouns people identify themselves with (she/her, he/him, they/them, ze/zir). It is not optional to call someone by their preferred pronoun—it is a required act of respect.

Queer: An umbrella term that encompasses all non-heterosexual and/or non-cisgender identities.

(Trans)gender: Someone who identifies with a gender other than their sex assigned at birth.

Two-spirit: An umbrella term used by First Nations people to recognize people who are a third gender (which is a blend of masculine and feminine energy), have multiple genders, or have identities that operate outside of the Western dichotomy of sex orientation and gender.

Note: *Female-bodied and male-bodied are commonly used terms that assume a body is within a binary, which is not true. Because there is not yet succinct language to talk about bodies outside of a binary context, in places I will be using this terminology with the understanding that the topic is far more complicated.*

Infinite Combinations

Sexuality, gender, sexual orientation, gender expression, and anatomy are a fluid part of human identity, which is becoming more and more fluid with each generation. All of these factors may shift throughout one's life, and any combination is possible.

SEXUALITY:

△ ASEXUAL

◩ DEMISEXUAL

◬ HOMOSEXUAL

▲ BISEXUAL

▲ PANSEXUAL

△ HETEROSEXUAL

GENDER:

◪ TRANSGENDER WOMAN OR TRANS WOMAN

◒ CISGENDER WOMAN OR CIS WOMAN

■ GENDERQUEER

⊡ NON-BINARY

□ AGENDER

◩ TRANSGENDER MAN OR TRANS MAN

⊟ CISGENDER MAN OR CIS MAN

GENDER EXPRESSION:

⊙ ANDROGYNOUS

◗ FEMININE

◖ MASCULINE

SEX:

⬟ FEMALE

⬠ MALE

⬟ INTERSEX

ATTRACTION:

☆ AROMANTIC

★ HOMOROMANTIC

✪ HETEROROMANTIC

✦ PANROMANTIC

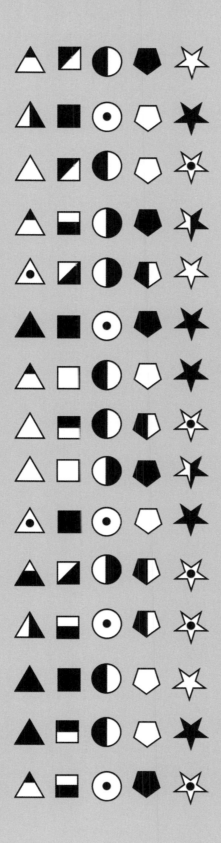

Gender Identity

Gender identity is our internal sense of self as a gender—who we know ourselves to be. A cisgender person has a gender identity that is consistent with the sex they were assigned at birth. A transgender or genderqueer person has a gender identity that is different than the sex they were assigned at birth.

EXAMPLES:

- Woman
- Man
- Agender
- Boy
- Non-binary
- Genderqueer

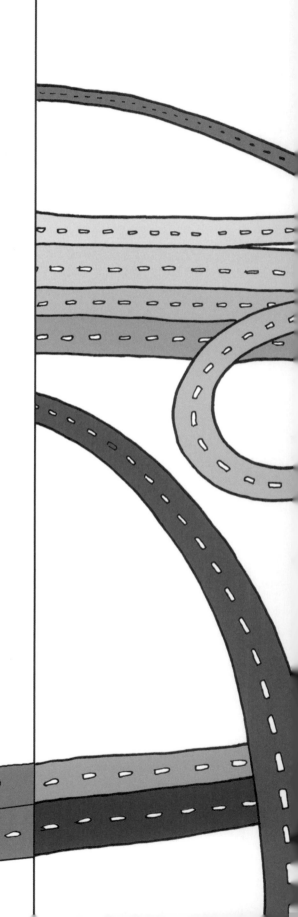

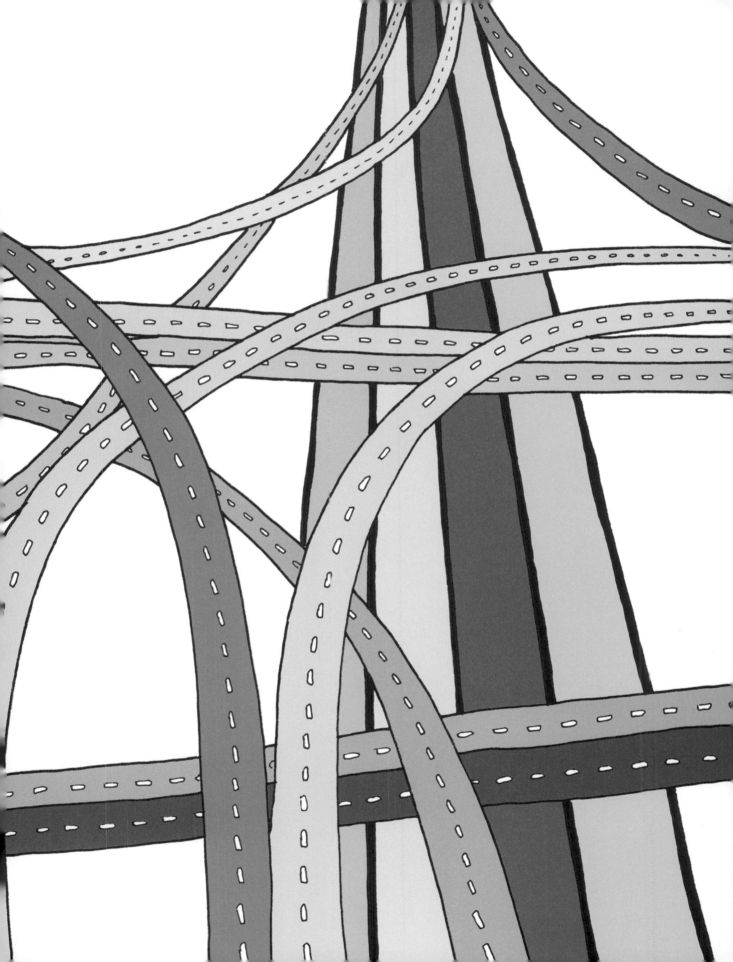

Pronouns: What They Are and Why They Matter

We use pronouns to describe each other all the time: she/her, he/him, they/them. Most people don't actively choose their pronouns, because they align with their gender identity by default.

For a cis woman, her sex is female, her gender is woman, and her pronoun is she/her.

For someone gender non-conforming, transgender, agender, or intersex, these assigned pronouns may not feel aligned with their gender identities. It's vital to respect someone's chosen pronoun and/or name (a former name no longer in use is often referred to as a *dead name*). Many people who are on the spectrum of gender or completely outside of she/he identities choose to use the gender-neutral they/them pronouns that replace she/her or he/him grammatically and in concept. The excuses of why people refuse to refer to someone in their life as a gender-neutral pronoun include:

- "It's too hard."
- "It's unnatural."
- "It's not that big of a deal."
- "It doesn't make sense grammatically, it's plural."

None of these are good or valid excuses to not try! Everyone will mess up in the beginning and that's okay; just making the effort indicates consideration and respect.

In response to those excuses, I would ask you to consider these points:

- It's really not too hard. We easily learn to call newlywed people by a new last name.
- Language evolves. This is an evolution of language.
- Everything feels "unnatural" at first but then becomes normalized. We created language, so we can change it.
- Think about if everyone in your life began calling you by pronouns different from your gender. You'd feel pretty bad, wouldn't you?
- Someone lost their wallet. There, you did it! You used a singular *they*.

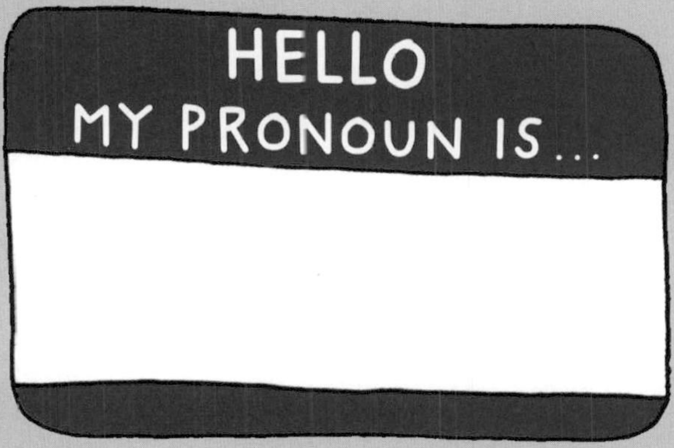

All of these people identify as non-binary.

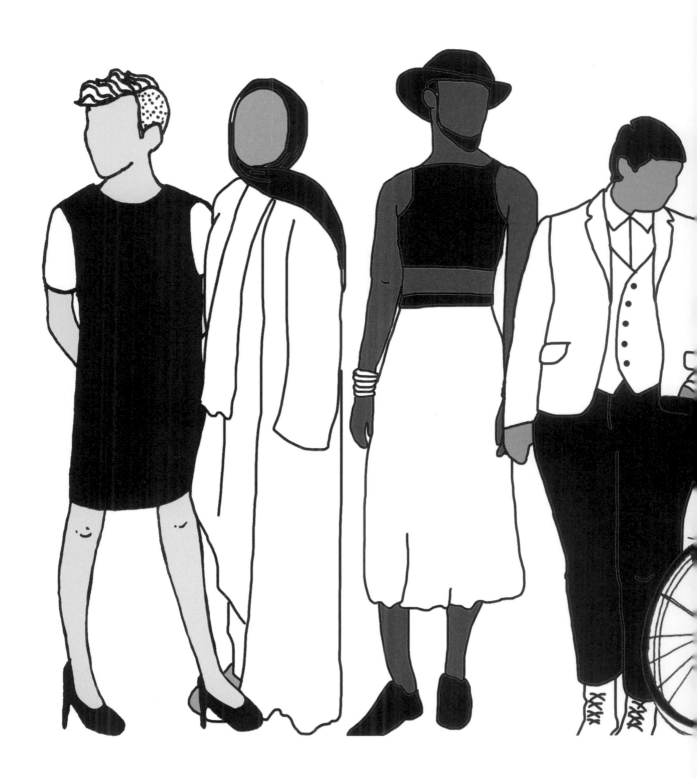

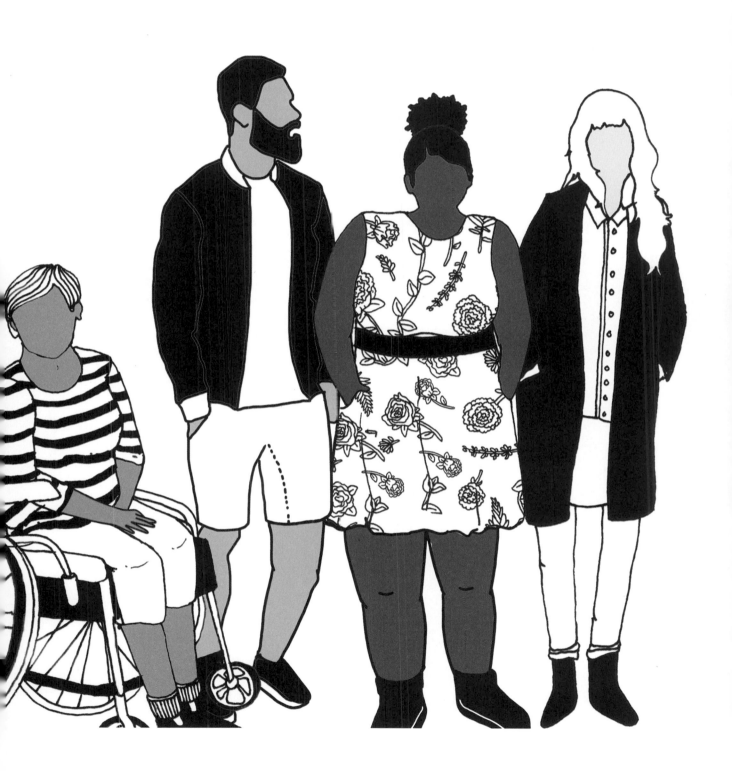

Spotlight on:

David Bowie (1947–2016)

"I don't know where I'm going from here, but I promise it won't be boring."

–DAVID BOWIE

David Bowie was known and idolized for his wild fashion, gender exploration, and musical legacy. A leader of the glam rock movement, Bowie embodied many personas throughout his life, most famously that of Ziggy Stardust, a fictional bisexual alien rock star, a flamboyant performer with bright hair, full makeup, and androgynous over-the-top costumes. Bowie consistently changed his personas, but no matter who he was at any moment, he was always Bowie.

He was the first superstar to completely shatter the mold of masculinity without it being directly tied to any specific sexual orientation. Bowie created a category of identity that was revolutionary in its fluidity and exploration of gender and sexuality. Dresses, face paint, glitter, onesies, bright hair, high heels, blouses, lipstick, silk scarves, gaudy jewelry—nothing was off-limits.

Both an entertainer and master of shape-shifting in music and fashion, his presence has had lasting effects on the creative world. Taking fashion elements from many cultures and eras, today's fashion—from Alexander McQueen to Lady Gaga to queer youth—shows his influence.

While Bowie made a huge impact on pop culture during his time and beyond, his legacy is complicated. Both before and after his death, women have either stated that Bowie engaged in sexual activity with them while they were minors (which constitutes statutory rape) or accused him of sexually assaulting them. Some of these women do not consider themselves to be victims of sexual assault and others do, but one thing is clear: he used his position of power to take advantage of young women. In the 1970s and '80s, celebrities were not often publicly held accountable for their misconduct, but we must now recognize the faults and wrong-doings of the idols held by popular culture. We can still hold Bowie as an icon of free expression and experimental music but should simultaneously acknowledge his harmful and unethical behavior.

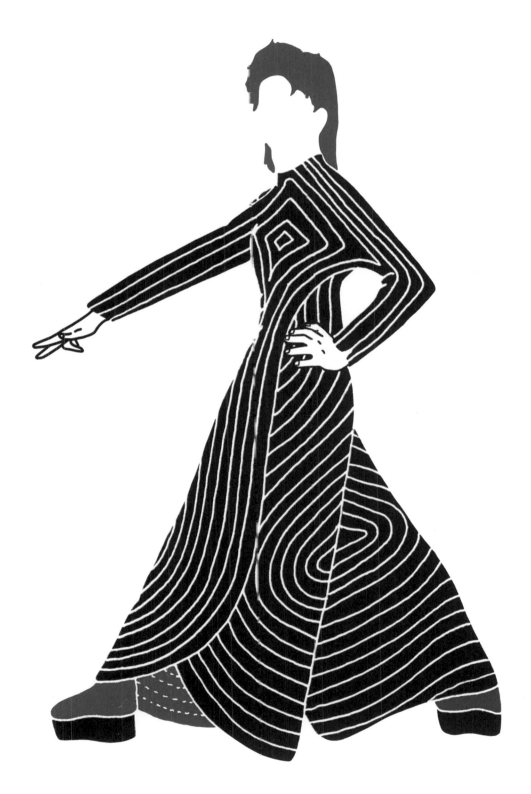

⌃ COSTUME BY KANSAI YAMAMOTO

Gender Dysphoria

Gender dysphoria is when your body doesn't feel in alignment with your gender identity.

One can feel uncomfortable socially, physically, or emotionally and may alleviate that discomfort by socially transitioning (changing pronouns or name), changing style, or physically changing through surgery or hormones. These are all important ways of achieving comfort in one's body.

If it's hard to imagine what that discomfort might feel like, do this thought experiment: You wake up one day to find you have the sexual characteristics, wardrobe, or gender roles of a gender you do not identify with. If you are a cisgender male, imagine having breasts, a menstrual cycle, or a feminine name. You might feel uncomfortable and ask people to respect you by calling you by a name that better suits your internal identity, or seek medical treatment to become masculine presenting.

There is a narrative that transgender people have always felt as if they've been trapped in the wrong body. While this is true for many people, oftentimes gender dysphoria develops and changes over time in a nonlinear fashion and is alleviated by one or more of the preceding options, but not all. Cisgender women can opt to have their breasts reduced, enlarged, or removed to feel more comfortable in their body while not shifting their gender identity. Female-assigned, gender-non-conforming people (born female but identifying as neither male nor female) can take testosterone hormones to develop secondary sex characteristics (facial hair, deepened voice, broad shoulders) but never use male pronouns. The needs and desires of someone to feel at home in themselves can vary widely. Changes can be made suddenly and in major ways or slowly in small increments, and **every iteration is valid and okay.**

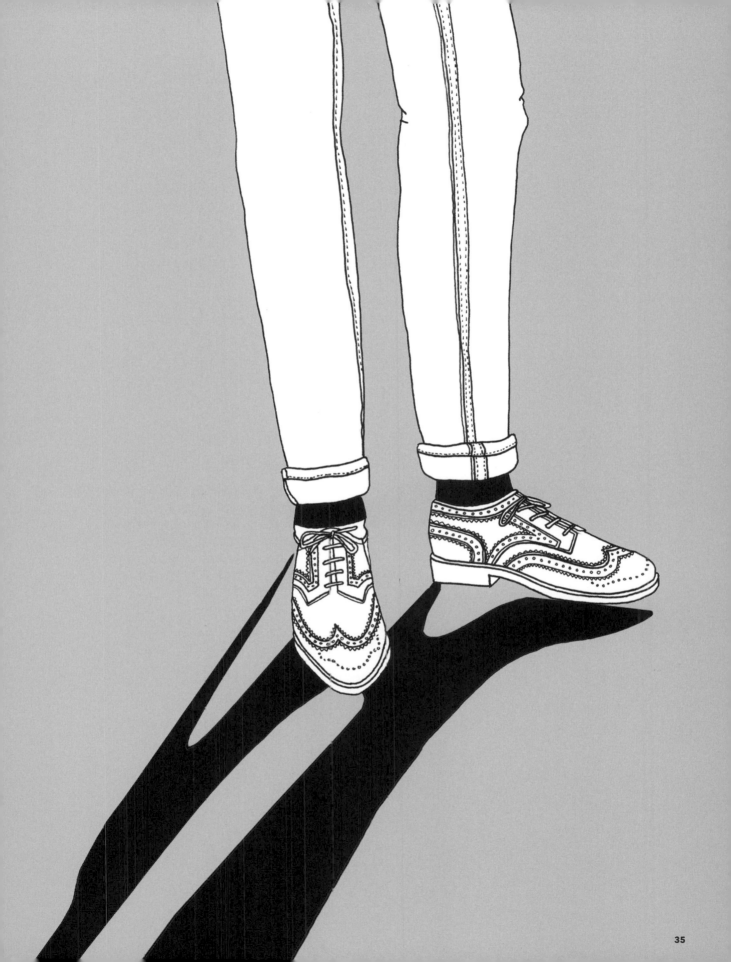

Children should be believed when they state they are a gender other than the sex they were assigned at birth.

And should be believed if they want to change their gender the next day.

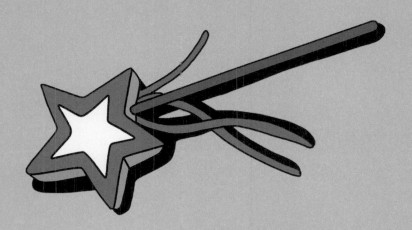

Gender Expression

Gender expression is deeply tied to traditional gender roles, division of labor, systems of oppression, and cultural norms. **Keep in mind that gender expression does not necessarily indicate gender identity!** For many reasons including (but not limited to) preference, comfort, safety, geographical location, and religion, someone's gender might not be presented in the social norm fashion of that gender. A boy living in a conservative town may not be able to present as feminine even though they wish to. A cisgender boy can wear dresses and still be a cisgender boy.

Some examples of how gender is expressed:

- High femme
- Androgynous
- Masculine
- Feminine
- Butch

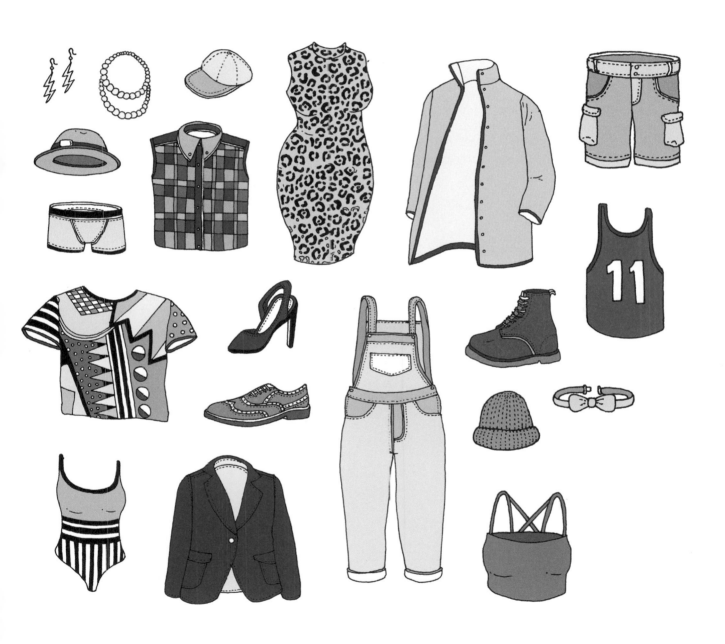

All of these items belong to one person's wardrobe.

The How, What, and Who of Attraction

The Difference Between Gender Identity, Sexual Orientation, and Sexuality

It can be really difficult to separate the three, as we often think of them as one thing. It's okay to be confused! A good exercise in thinking about these as distinct elements is to assess your own landscape of attraction.

1. What's your gender identity? Cisgender woman, transgender boy, genderqueer, or not sure yet?

2. Who are you attracted to? Everyone? Someone of the same gender as you or different? Not attracted to anyone?

3. How do you like to be intimate or in relationships with people? Monogamous? No sex at all? Several romantic partners? And what happens behind closed doors (or open, if you're into that) with the person you're attracted to?

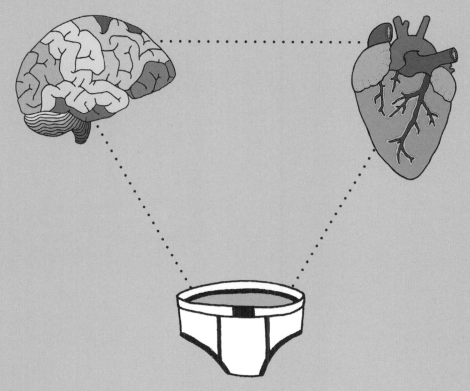

GENDER IDENTITY IS THE **SELF**
(INTERNAL UNDERSTANDING)

SEXUAL ORIENTATION IS THE **WHO** OF DESIRE
(EXTERNAL DESIRE FOR OTHERS)

SEXUALITY IS THE **HOW** AND **WHAT** OF DESIRE
(HOW YOU LIKE TO BE INTIMATE)

Spotlight on:

Prince (1958–2016)

"I'm not a woman / I'm not a man / I am something that you'll never understand."

—"I WOULD DIE 4 U"

I love Prince in all his eccentric purple glory. His given name was actually Prince (full name: Prince Rogers Nelson), after his father's jazz stage name, a name fit for someone who would become one of the top-selling musical artists in history and a fashion icon of the twentieth century.

Prince was a musical genius and an incredibly prolific artist (forty-two albums and vaults full of unreleased music), but when we think of Prince, we think of his colorful, flamboyant, unapologetically androgynous, and wildly sexual presence. He showed the world a different expression of Blackness as one of the most gender-fluid performers to date. He defied the confines of race, sexuality, gender, and fashion, wearing wild outfits and eyeliner and possessing an air of mystery. At one point, he changed his name to an unpronounceable symbol, a mash-up of the gender symbols for man and woman plus some added flair. He was a Black man who proudly and confidently embraced the masculine and feminine within himself. He broke all the rules.

Prince was full of complexity and contradiction and perfectly demonstrated the distinction between gender identity and sexual orientation. He was a straight feminine man and both a queer/transgender icon and a conservative Jehovah's Witness. His complexity forces us to challenge the assumptions we hold about the intersection of gender, sexuality, and religion.

Later in his life (after he'd become a Jehovah's Witness), he gave a few interviews in which he seemed to be antigay. His former bandmates Wendy Melvoin and Lisa Coleman said that he asked them to denounce their homosexuality before he'd play with them again. However, several years later they performed on the same stage.

How can a gay icon be against queerness? How can a pioneer in freedom of sexual expression be straight?

Well that's just it: People are complex and ever shifting. One category never automatically means another. Regardless of his political or spiritual beliefs later in life, Prince paved the way for people to feel freer in their expression of identity.

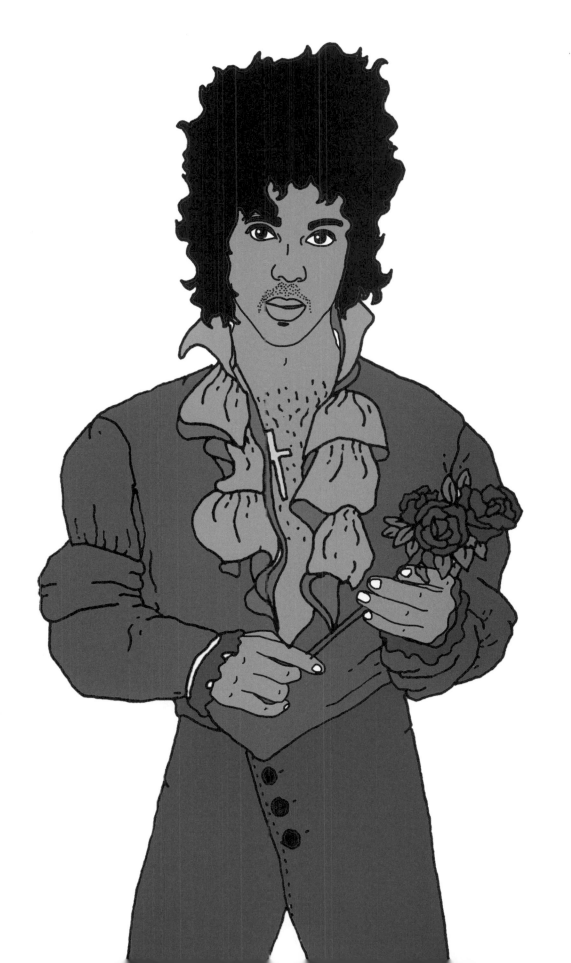

Asexuality

Asexuality isn't talked about too much, but it should be!

Asexuality is a sexual orientation in which people do not experience much (if any) sexual attraction and have a low or absent desire for sexual activity. Unlike celibacy, it's not a choice, and has nothing to do with romantic or sexual orientation (who you're attracted to). Much like the term queer, asexuality is an umbrella term under which many types of more specific orientations fall. **Just like any other facet of identity, sexuality is on a fluid spectrum.** One might experience sexual attraction only if they feel an emotional connection (demisexual) or have romantic attraction without the sexual component. Most people who identify as asexual maintain that identity consistently, even if they are in a relationship long term, though some people shift in and out of periods of asexuality.

I have, at times, identified as asexual, so it's very important to me that this topic be included in this book. There is almost no representation of asexuals in popular media and it's often not believed to be a real orientation, so I want to give it attention and representation. Having no interest in sex is shamed in American culture, making it very hard for people to come out as asexual. Because of this, there can be a lot of internalized shame and feelings of inherent brokenness.

People often try to convince asexual people that they aren't, attributing it to past trauma, or firing off any number of backhanded compliments or blatant insults. For future reference, don't say any of the following to an asexual person:

- "Maybe you haven't been with the right person." (Irrelevant.)
- "Don't be a prude." (I'm not.)
- "That's not real." (Yes, it is.)
- "It's just a phase." (Nope, it's my sexuality.)

- "You never know until you try." (Yeah, I do know.)
- "Don't you mean celibate?" (No, that's a choice.)
- "What about kids?" (There are other ways to have kids, and it's fine if I don't want them.)
- "You probably just had a bad experience once." (Irrelevant, or I had a bad experience because I thought I was supposed to want to have sex. Sometimes trauma can affect sexuality, but asexuality as related to trauma is still asexuality, and its validity should not be questioned.)

It's so important to trust people when they express this identity and support them in what might be a potentially difficult experience. Disbelief and shame from others can lead people to put themselves in uncomfortable sexual situations out of perceived social obligation or pressure, or avoid romantic relationships completely for fear of eventual rejection.

Asexuality can also be really great! There is absolutely no limit to how romantic and loving relationships can be with someone who is asexual. There are so many ways to be intimate without sex. With sex off the table, there is more time for reading, walking, seeing friends, exploring other interests, and maybe a bit more free space in your brain for things that make you happy and fulfilled. Asexual people are just like sexual people in that not all of them want to be in a relationship.

Asexuality is not a lack or a deficiency of something valuable—it's just a different sexuality. You're not less valuable than another person with a different sexuality! You're important, and you are not alone!

Go gle

asexuality is |

asexuality is **wrong**
asexuality is **not lgbt**
asexuality is **not normal**
asexuality is **a disease**
asexuality is **a lie**
asexuality is **impossible**
asexuality is **a choice**
asexuality is **a spectrum**
asexuality is **normal**

Report inappropriate predictions

*ACTUAL GOOGLE SUGGESTIONS

Homosexual Behavior in Animals

It's debatable whether animals have sexualities (sexual preferences or attractions outside of the survival instinct to procreate). A huge number of animal species have been observed engaging in mating behavior—not necessarily sexual behavior—with individuals of the same sex. There are many explanations for this: expression of dominance, courting behavior, nonsexual partnership, affection, or stimulating reproductive hormones without a viable mate.

Here are a few of the many species that exhibit frequent same-sex behavior or have long-term, same-sex partners: black swans, dragonflies, elephants, bats, whiptail lizards, hyenas, penguins, cows, giraffes, dolphins, and marmots. Bonobo apes are, as a species, almost entirely bisexual and engage regularly in nonreproductive sex with both males and females. By the way, humans evolved from apes, and most ape species are very sexually fluid . . . just sayin'.

Ten percent of male rams will exclusively mate with other male sheep, even in the presence of ewes (the opportunity to carry on their genes).

There's nothing unnatural about it.

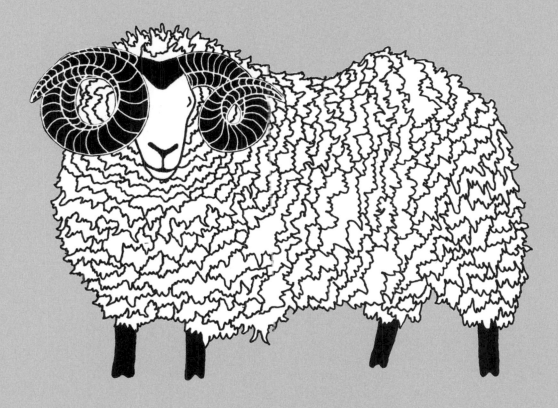

⌃ A GAY RAM

Physical Sex

Physical sex is the physical, biological makeup of one's reproductive organs, chromosomes, hormones, and secondary sex characteristics (facial and body hair, vocal range, breasts).

When a baby is born, the doctor looks at their genitalia and decides what gender the baby will be raised as. This is not a very precise science and doesn't consider many of the other factors that contribute to one's physical sex characteristics. This process can be very damaging to intersex people (see page 50).

Many people believe sex (unlike gender) is immutable, which is not true. Sex is not binary, but a spectrum. For example, not all men have lots of facial hair and deep voices, and not all women have wide hips and lack facial hair.

Much like one's gender presentation, sex can shift over time. One can also make changes to their sex through surgery or hormones.

Anatomy of Gender

Unbounded possibility of imagination, vulnerability, brilliance, creativity, anger, love, and complexity.

Upper lip hair is common in female-bodied people.

Facial and body hair is affected by testosterone levels and can be altered (decreased or increased) with hormone therapy. Trans men can grow beards, and people with biologically male-dominant traits can remain relatively hairless their whole lives. Cisgender women also have testosterone.

Vocal range and presence of an Adam's apple. Vocal range changes with puberty or hormone therapy.

There is a great range in natural breast size and shape among female-bodied people. Some have had breast tissue removed to align with their appropriate gender, to alleviate discomfort, or due to illness like breast cancer. Male-bodied people also have breast tissue, and they can also get breast cancer. Female-bodied people may have breast implants to align more with their gender.

Hip width is generally greater in bodies that have uteruses for childbirth.

Genitalia and reproductive organs do not always reflect chromosomes, hormones, or gonads. Genitals can be changed by surgery and hormone blockers. Many male- and female-bodied people have had their gonads (internal sexual organs, ovaries or testicles) removed for medical reasons, such as ovarian or testicular cancer. Sex organs are not determinant of one's gender.

Body hair is often thought of as a male trait, but all humans (and all mammals, even dolphins) have body hair. Many female-bodied people have more body hair than male-bodied people. Female hairlessness is a white beauty standard, bringing shame to women of color, who tend to have more body hair.

Intersex

There is a fundamental problem in the way society—and particularly, doctors—determine the sex (and therefore assumed gender) of babies at birth. The practice of sex assignment of newborns has been strictly female or male. The binary is still upheld in most societies worldwide, including in the United States. If a baby is born intersex (has some sort of genital or gonadal structure that varies from strict definitions of female or male bodies), it is considered "abnormal"; someone (usually a doctor) chooses a sex, and the baby either has surgery or is prescribed hormones (or both) to make them "match" the assigned sex. This amounts to nonconsensual gender reassignment surgery, unethical genital mutilation, and possible sterilization for thousands of children born with non-binary genitals.

Intersex children forced into a binary sex are having someone else determine what their body will be before they're allowed to grow into their gender identity. As they grow older, they may experience, at best, limited access to appropriate health care because of their unique situation or, at worst, discrimination, stigmatization, or even murder.

Because this subject is so taboo, people assume that being intersex is a rare occurrence, but it is actually quite common. The following statistics from the study "How Sexually Dimorphic Are We?," by Anne Fausto-Sterling et al., show that the variation and rate of non-binary sexual characteristics is vast and common. Note: This is a very small sample of the huge variation of ways to be intersex.

Numbers of intersex births are always debated (because definitions of what makes a baby "intersex" are not standardized) and change dramatically depending on what article you read, but these numbers are supported by the Intersex Society of North America and American Psychological Association:

Total number of people:

- Whose bodies differ from standard male or female = 1 in 100 births
- Who have visibly atypical genitalia = 1 in 1,500 births
- Who receive surgery to "normalize" genital appearance = 1 or 2 in 1,000 births
- Who don't have XX or XY chromosomes (such as a female with only one X or someone who has XXY chromosomes) = 1 in 1,666 births

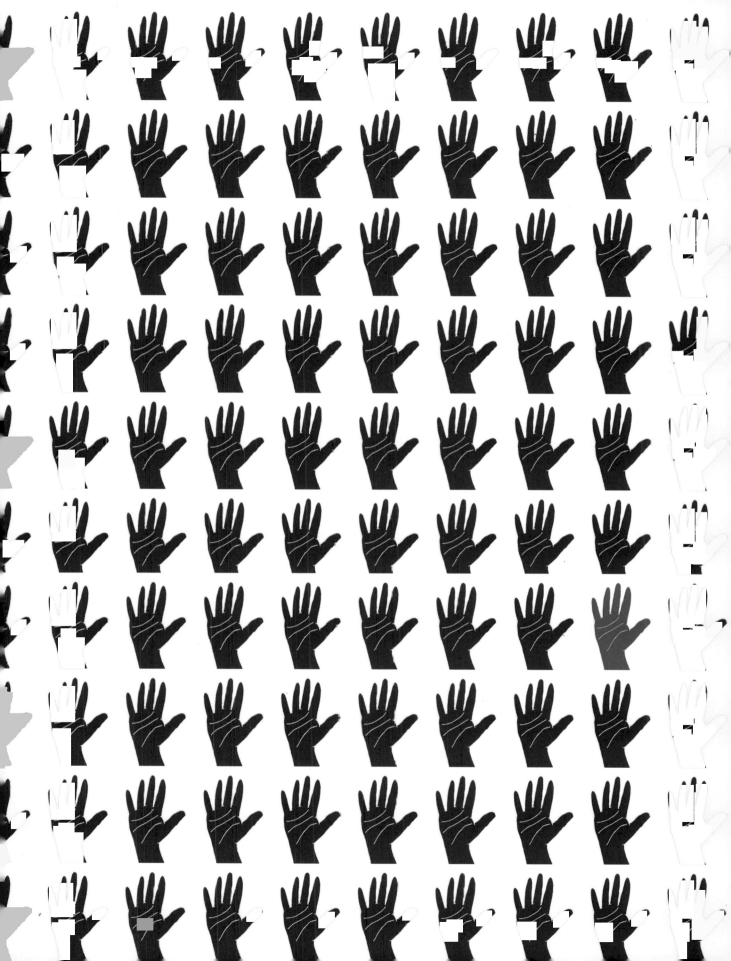

Slug Sex

We've all seen a slug—and have possibly stepped on one. Slimy, slow, and squishy, these shell-less terrestrial gastropod mollusks also have one of the most sexually fluid existences. Slugs are hermaphroditic, meaning they have both male and female reproductive organs. This common trait among invertebrates and plants gives them an evolutionary advantage: Any individual of a species can mate with any other individual. If there are no available partners, the individual can fertilize themselves!

Terminology note: While the term *hermaphrodite* is outdated and offensive when used to refer to human beings (intersex is the appropriate term), the word is still acceptable to use when referring to nonhuman species. Sexual polymorphism also describes species with both sexual organs.

When two leopard slugs (or any slugs) find each other in the wild, they will entangle in a slimy spiral, hanging upside down to exchange spermatozoa.

The evolutionary ingenuity of sexual polymorphism is that in addition to being able to give and receive sperm, both individuals possess eggs. They can fertilize each other's eggs, producing twice the number of offspring while simultaneously achieving genetic variation.

If something goes . . . um, wrong, the slugs will become stuck in their tangled state, and a sacrifice must be made to get free: One of the slugs must bite off the male organ of the other. Because the now-amputated slug retains its female reproductive organs, luckily it can continue to mate and reproduce with other individuals that have male organs.

Slugs who don't find a mate can fertilize their own eggs with their own sperm, resulting in viable (but less genetically diverse) offspring.

Don't underestimate the humble slug.

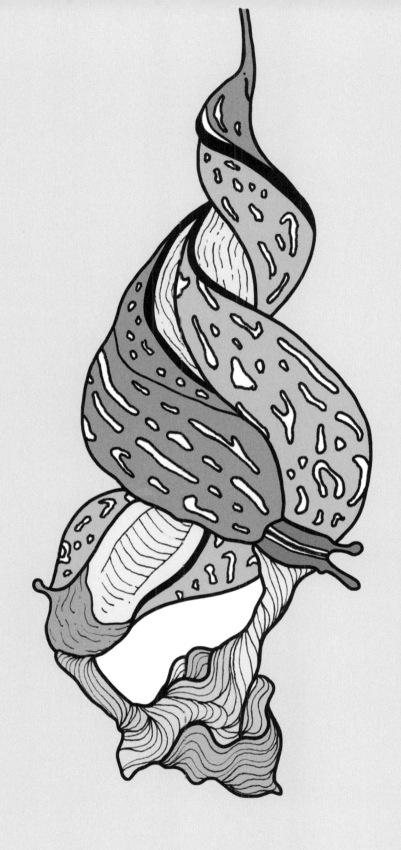

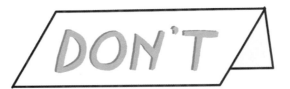

DON'T

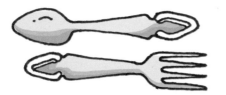

DON'T ask someone's birth name!

DON'T give backhanded compliments! ("But your name is so pretty!" "You're too pretty to be gay!")

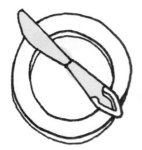

DON'T misgender someone behind their back.

DON'T make someone else's gender about you. If you feel uncomfortable, spend time processing it on your own, with friends, or in therapy.

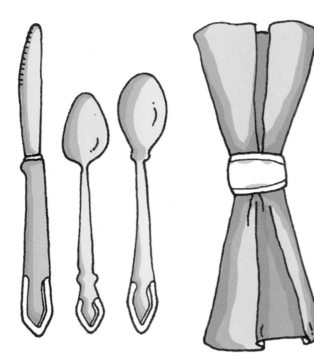

DON'T comment on people's bodies (particularly if someone's body is changing). It is only appropriate if the person initiates the topic themselves.

DON'T see it as a threat to your appearance or presentation if you're cisgender and are asked your pronoun. It's just a question, not an implication!

DON'T be mean!

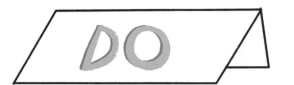

DO be patient with people's processes! Everyone moves at their own speed.

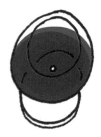

DO trust that people select the bathroom that makes them feel safe and is in line with their gender. Don't assume you know better than they do.

PRACTICE MAKES ~~PERFECT~~ PROGRESS

DO ask people's pronouns even if you think their gender is obvious. Sometimes gender expressions and identity are different! While it's not relevant to some people, it's really important to others and is a small, meaningful, quick gesture everyone can do.

DO be nice!

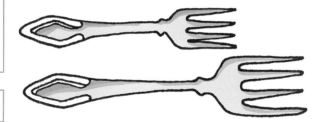

What Does LGBTQ+ Actually Mean?

When I was once asked why there is no S for straight in the acronym LGBTQ+, it made me realize that maybe the phrase isn't fully understood by those outside of the community it describes. The intention of LGBTQ+ is to describe everyone who is not cisgender and/or straight. Including S defeats the entire purpose of the acronym! Over the years, the acronym has evolved as letters have been added and the phrase is used in different ways.

A brief history of how LGBTQ+ came to be the accepted term:

- **Pre-1950s:** The most common descriptor was *homosexual*, which was used in a derogatory manner to describe anyone non-straight. *Gay* began to be used as a slang term in the 1940s and '50s.

- **1950s-1960s:** *Homosexual* was replaced with *homophile*.

- **1970s-1980s:** During this time, there was conflict within the LGBTQ+ community for categorical recognition both from the outside world and within the community. Self-identified lesbians demanded visibility, which shifted the terminology away from homophile and toward gay and lesbian, while queer was still used as a derogatory and often dangerous insult. The B and T of LGBT were not recognized at this time, and transgender and bisexual people were (and often still are) harmfully ostracized and excluded from the LGBTQ+ community by those within it. Bisexual people were viewed as dishonest—that they were fearful of being openly or "fully" gay.

- **1990s:** LGBT was widely accepted as a term of inclusivity. In 1996, Q was added for queer (or questioning), to form the acronym we most commonly use now. Black human rights activist Cleo Manago coined the term SGL (same-gender-loving) to describe the African American population's experience as separate from the more Eurocentric gay and lesbian. The term AGL (all-gender-loving) has also been accepted as a positive identity within the Black community. While those terms are embraced by some, many African Americans don't identify with SGL or AGL. They don't believe the word gay has inherently white ownership, yet they recognize that racism in the gay community needs to be acknowledged.

- **2000s-2010s:** This decade saw the phasing out of *gay* used as a slur from popular vocabulary. Younger people tend to identify more strongly with the term *queer*, as it allows room for much more fluidity of gender and sexuality. While it's increasingly a more comfortable term for this generation, many older people have a negative reaction to it due to their experiences with the word as a slur in their youth.

- **2010s-2020s:** Language around gender and sexuality expanded significantly as acceptance and visibility of LGBTQ+ people has grown. In large part because of the internet, access to information has become easier and a wider variety of voices can be heard. More people in the United States identify as LGBTQ+ than ever before, with 5.6% of Americans identifying as LGBTQ+ in 2021 versus 4.5% in 2017. Whether this is because people are coming to understand their own sexuality more or that it's safer to be out is unclear, but either way, the visibility and conversation around issues of identity are becoming more common and acceptable.

Some variations on the acronym include additional letters (such as I for intersex) or drop some for a plus sign to signify the expansiveness of gender and sexuality identities. Some people switch around the order of the letters to signify different emphases on certain groups. To show how infinite the realms of gender and sexuality are, there is a lengthy acronym: LGBTTQQIAAP (lesbian, gay, bisexual, transgender, transsexual, queer, questioning, intersex, asexual, ally, pansexual). There is heavy debate (mostly from allies themselves) about whether A should include ally, as this is not necessarily someone who identifies as not straight and/or not cisgender and implies that supporting queer people means falling under the umbrella of the queer community. I personally do not agree with its inclusion and hope allies will be allies regardless of being overtly labeled as such. It's important for the queer community to be recognized and be supported without symbolic applause (being included in the acronym).

Another acronym (which is by far the funniest) is QUILTBAG (queer and questioning, undecided, intersex, lesbian, transgender and two-spirit, bisexual, asexual and ally. and gay and genderqueer). Both of these long acronyms highlight the fact that no acronym will ever encompass every experience one could have. Most people prefer to use the shorter LGBTQ+ and infer that it includes the spectrum of experience within it. However, people continue to feel excluded by the acronym, which is why this text fluctuates between using LGBTQ+ and LGBTQIA+. It's quite possible there will be another permutation in the near future as understandings of gender and sexuality continue to evolve.

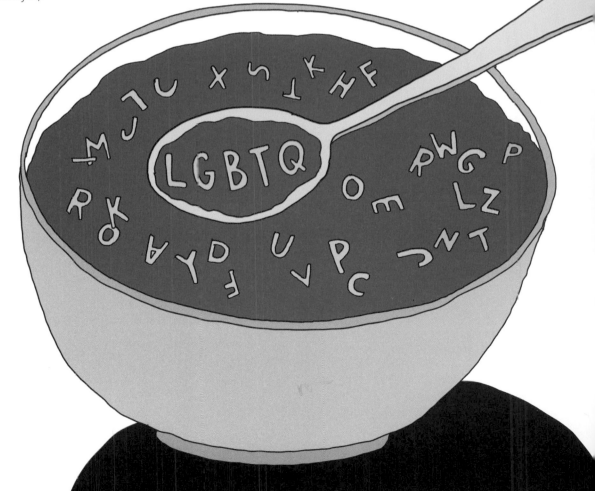

Gender Roles: The Parts We Were Cast to Play

Gender roles are expectations about behavior, appearance, communication style, demeanor, and work based on assigned sex. There are similar manifestations of gender roles across countries, cultures, races, religions, and time. However, there are also variations in and deviations from masculinity, femininity, and the associated roles of the two within and between cultures.

Let's get one thing out of the way: **All gender roles have been socially created.** We made them. Some behavior, tendencies, and traits are strongly biologically influenced depending on the sex of a person, but they are rarely, if ever, a reason behind enforcing gender roles.

These gender constructs do not properly reflect the true abundance of intelligence, power, and autonomy of women, or the emotional potential, gentleness, and nurturing qualities of men. Everyone is a complicated soup of human traits, interests, skills, and expression, but society doesn't allow for much wiggle room outside of traditional gender roles or provide many role models for those who want to break away from expected behaviors.

Gender stereotypes (alongside race, ability, and socioeconomic factors) have contributed to the rise in toxic masculinity, a culture rampant with sexual assault, enormous pay wage gaps, male-dominated governmental control of women's reproductive rights, and a media culture that portrays mainly heteronormative models of relationships and gender.

Relationships between gay men, as well as between butch and femme women, are expected to hold distinct gender roles and divisions of labor, such as expecting the butch partner to have a gruffer personality and be less vulnerable, and for the femme partner to do the emotional heavy lifting. "So, who wears the pants?" or "Which one is the bride?" are quintessential questions that sum this up—they assume one of the two women must be closer to a man, or one of the two men must be more feminine to be in a functional relationship.

"When are you going to have kids?" is one of the top questions asked of heterosexual relationships. The woman is expected to want children, and if she has them, she is expected to be the primary caregiver while the dad is available only for fun weekend times or discipline. On the flip side, this gender assumption often leaves fathers without equivalent paternity leave, increasing the need for women to take time off from work while reinforcing the idea of a more absent father figure. However, if the father does provide more than the absolute minimum of childcare and/or house upkeep, he's given high praise (while women receive no praise at all for doing the same things).

Male bosses are expected to be firm, tough, and stern as a measure of career success and power, while women in powerful positions displaying the same characteristics are thought of as bossy.

Gender roles are applied in childhood. We're told how to act. Girls are supposed to be sweet and nice; boys aren't supposed to cry. We saw our gender role modeled in the adults around us (our parents, our teachers) and in all forms of media, so of course we tended to emulate it, were expected to fulfill it, and have come to expect it for ourselves.

Humans really like categories. We make them all the time—it helps things feel ordered and simple. It can be really difficult to break from the expectations of what you should be, based on what you look like. **It can be painful or mundane—but sometimes revolutionary.**

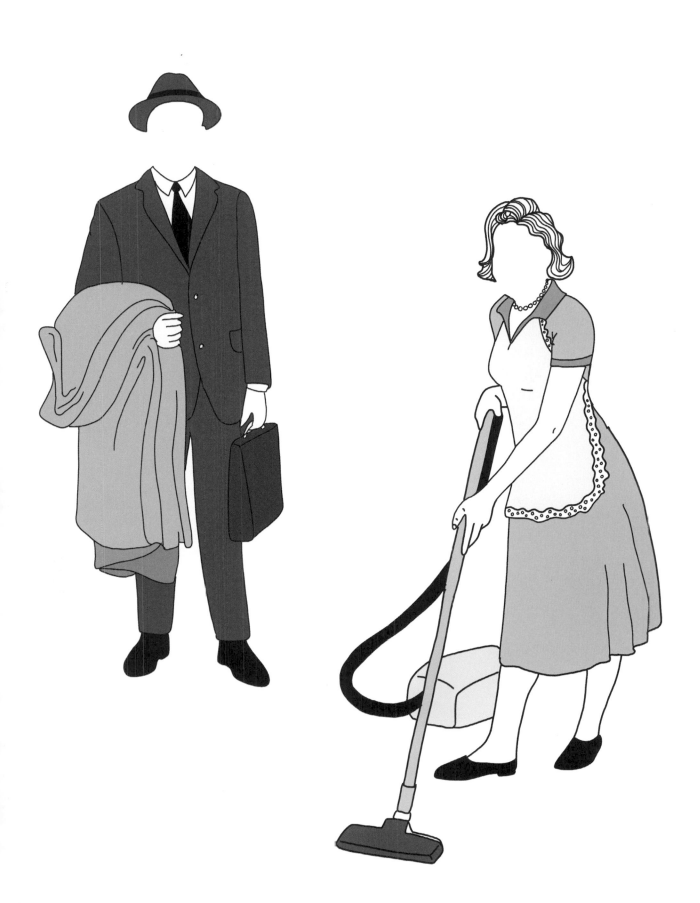

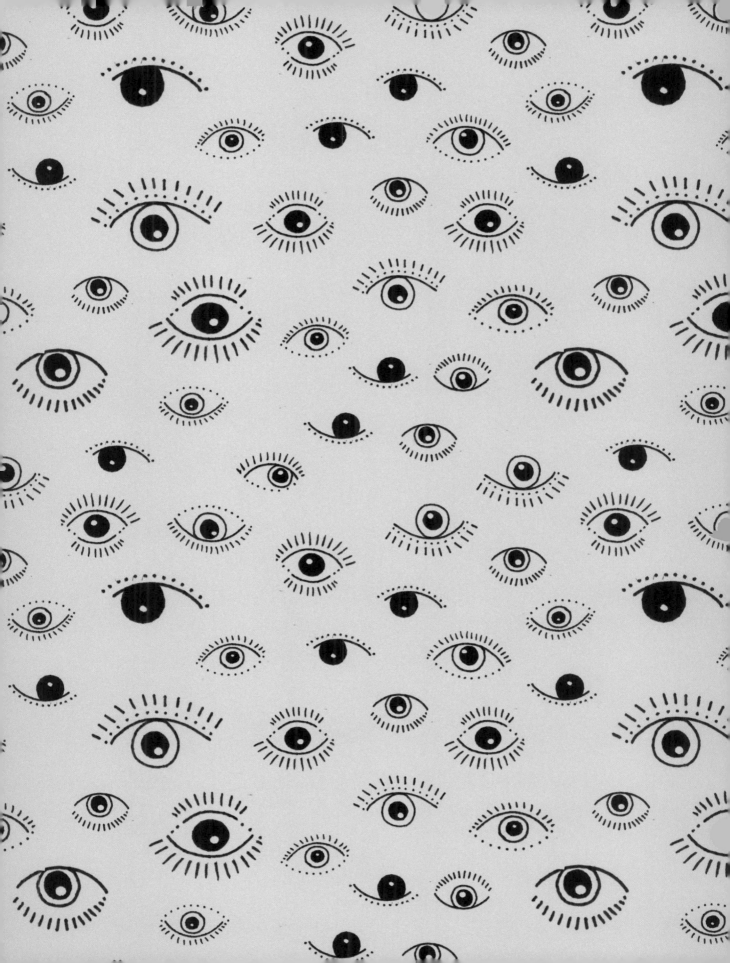

Digging Deeper

Intersectionality

"In every generation and in every intellectual sphere and in every political movement, there have been African American women who have articulated the need to think and talk about race through a lens that looks at gender, or think and talk about feminism through a lens that looks at race."

—DR. KIMBERLÉ CRENSHAW

Intersectionality is a term that has existed since the late 1980s, coined by Dr. Kimberlé Crenshaw, professor and civil rights advocate. The term was originally created to describe and study the lives of Black women and the ways in which their systemic disadvantages are not defined just by their womanhood, but by their Blackness. Crenshaw states, "The term was used to capture the applicability of Black feminism to antidiscrimination law."

The intersectional theory, in short, studies how different power structures interact to affect the lives of minorities. It highlights how each person is complex and multidimensional, and how those factors can combine to form systemic oppression and erasure. **One's experience in life is never isolated to only one sector of their identity;** they're not just their gender or race; their experience is an intersection of identities that lead to more or less privilege or oppression. The experiences of an elderly Black woman and a young Latino man in the same neighborhood will be completely different.

Intersectionality serves to highlight how marginalized members of certain populations are erased—such as women's movements that do not include trans women, or HIV/AIDS movements that do not show people of color. **As much as intersectionality illuminates oppression, it also reveals the populations with the most privilege.** This insight is important, as it is often harder to recognize our own privilege than to recognize the oppression of others. For a more thorough explanation of privilege, see page 136.

This book looks at gender from an intersectional perspective to explore why it is important to take all facets of a person into account when discussing the concept and experience of gender.

In short, things are more complicated than they seem.

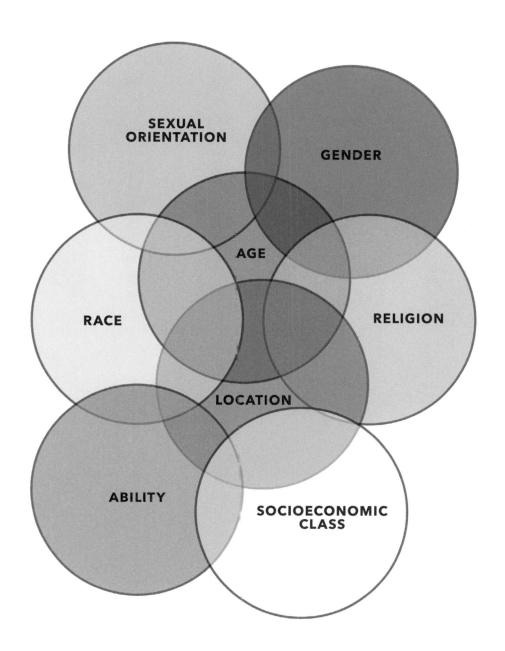

SEXUAL ORIENTATION

GENDER

AGE

RACE

RELIGION

LOCATION

ABILITY

SOCIOECONOMIC CLASS

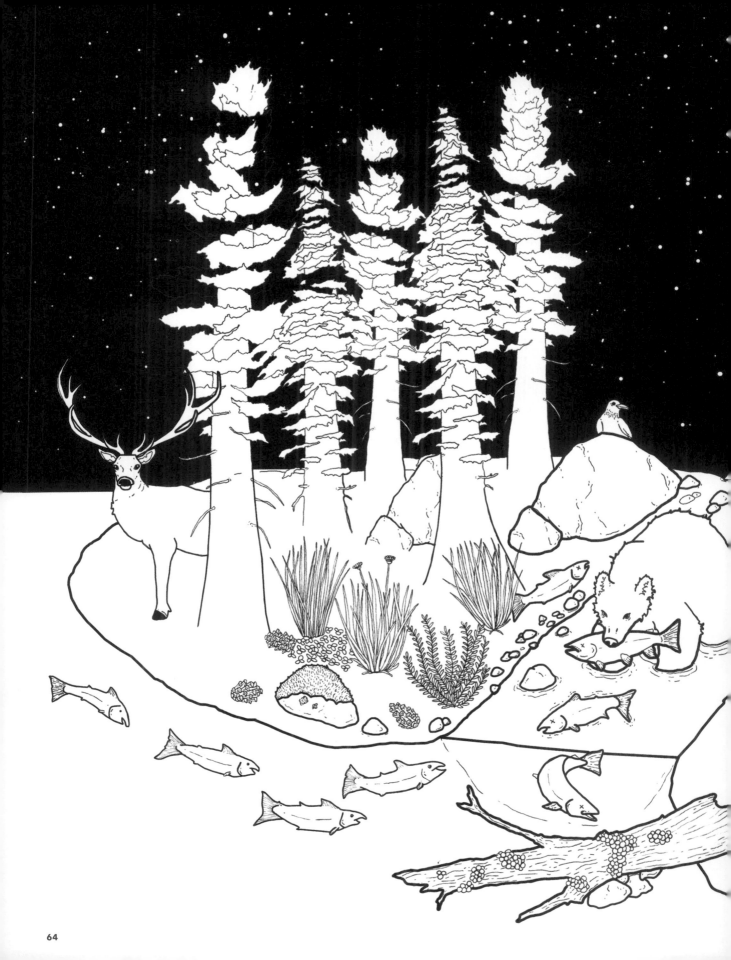

An Ecosystem of Identities Collapsed into Two

How Colonization in North America Imposed a Strong Gender Binary

"We define 'othering' as a set of dynamics, processes, and structures that engender marginality and persistent inequality across any of the full range of human differences based on group identities."

—JOHN A. POWELL AND STEPHEN MENENDIAN

Let's rewind. If we think about the root causes of sexism, misogyny, racism, classism, ageism, ableism, and all the -isms in this country, they are all about pretty much two things: othering and power. If we seek out the root of many of those dynamics, we will find that colonialism and imperialism brought an "othering" mentality to so much of the world and with it brought the gender binary.

"Colonization itself was a gendered act, carried out by imperial workforces, overwhelmingly men, drawn from masculinized occupations such as soldiering and long-distance trade. The rape of women of colonized societies was a normal part of conquest. The colonial state was built as a power structure operated by men, based on continuing force. Brutality was built into colonial societies."

—RAEWYN CONNELL, AUSTRALIAN SOCIOLOGIST

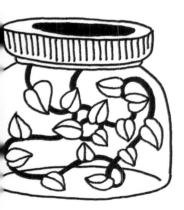
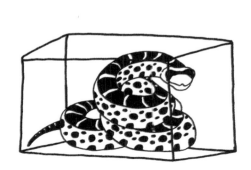
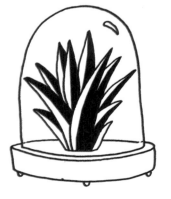
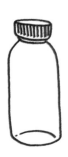

Most Native American cultures existed within their own systems of equity between themselves and the natural world. When colonists arrived in North America, they imposed the notion of hierarchy: humans above nature, whites above non-whites, men above women. When the European model of power was imposed on Indigenous peoples, a model in which wealthy white men exclusively held the decision- and law-making power, gender roles were automatically and simultaneously imposed upon them as well. Even though many Native American women held the highest positions of leadership in spiritual matters, governing, and families within their communities, they were seen as subordinate to men.

"That we do not fit easily into preexisting, officially recognized categories is the correlative of our culture of origin. . . . Neither does our thought fit the categories that have been devised to organize Western intellectual enterprise."
–PAULA GUNN ALLEN, FIRST NATIONS SCHOLAR

»FACING PAGE: LOZEN OF THE APACHE TRIBE—A WOMAN WARRIOR WHO FOUGHT TO PROTECT THE APACHE PEOPLE WITH HER REVERED AND MAGICAL SKILL OF LOCATING THREATENING ENEMIES—SURROUNDED BY NATIVE FAUNA AND FLORA OF NORTH AMERICA

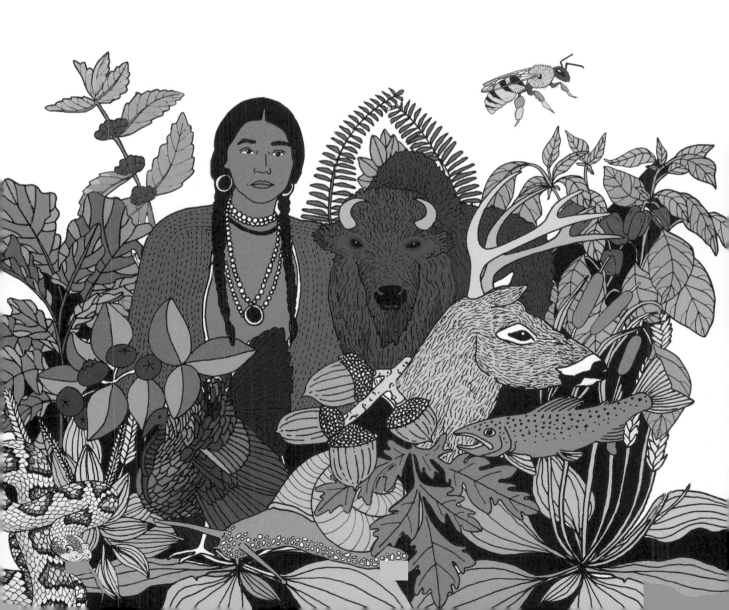

"*Strong as a man, braver than most and cunning in strategy, Lozen is a shield to her people.*"
–VICTORIO, AN APACHE CHIEF

Residential Schools

"The dehumanization suffered by our elders and our communities in the residential schools has had an intergenerational effect on aboriginal communities, and especially on two-spirited members of the community. The association of two-spiritedness with sin, and the erasure/denial of their very existence is the dominant culture/colonizer speaking with the voices of our elders."

–MICHELLE CAMERON, AUTHOR OF "TWO-SPIRITED ABORIGINAL PEOPLE: CONTINUING CULTURAL APPROPRIATION BY NON-ABORIGINAL SOCIETY"

In the 1880s, Canada created a system of boarding schools and later required that Indigenous, First Nations children attend a mandatory "residence school" in an effort to assimilate them into Christian European white culture. The government's intention was to put as much linguistic, familial, geographic, and cultural distance between the children and their native cultures as possible in order to gain systemic dominance. Stripping children of their traditions and languages at a young age left the younger generation in a cultural limbo, making it difficult for them to either reintegrate into their own culture or fully enter Eurocentric culture.

Attendance in these schools was an incredibly abusive and traumatic experience, and created a strong, divisive gender binary that did not previously exist in most Indigenous cultures. Cindy Hanson, former president of the Canadian Research Institute for the Advancement of Women, writes, "The Indian residential school system was, like other colonization programs . . . purposefully gendered to undermine and remove indigenous women's traditional authority, agency, and roles within families, clans, and traditional governance systems."

Women learned to be subservient as men took on more patriarchal roles in the family, often being more in control and having more decision-making power. Children were raised in nuclear family structures rather than in extended families and community. In many cases, two-spirit identities were damaged or lost in the process of forced assimilation. Communities that were taught to have certain prejudices now have to relearn how to revive other gender identities within the community.

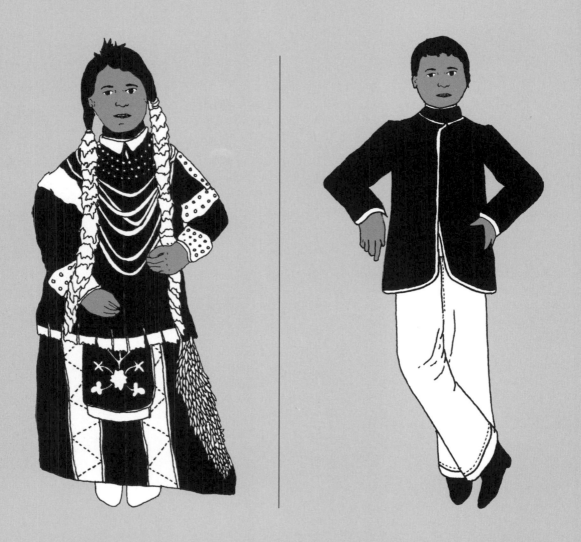

⌃THOMAS MOORE KEESICK BEFORE AND AFTER ENTERING THE REGINA INDIAN INDUSTRIAL SCHOOL

Third and Fourth Genders

Non-binary and other systems of categorizing genders are nothing new: third, fourth, and even fifth and sixth genders have existed in many cultures, for thousands of years in some cases. Almost every country has had a group of non-binary people. Some groups are revered as being spiritual leaders, shamans, or healers; others are ostracized or seen as outcasts within society.

A brief tour around the world of gender variance:

- **Il femminiello, Italy:** A third gender of men who are gendered as women but who do not identify as trans women or gay men. They are warmly accepted and are said to bring good luck to the families they were born into.

- **Muxe, Zapotec culture, Oaxaca, Mexico:** People assigned male at birth (AMAB) who identify as other genders. The expression and gender roles of muxe people vary widely. Muxe are respected and celebrated within their communities (but generally not outside of them).

- **Makkunrai, Oroané, Calabai, Calalai, and Bissu:** The five genders of the Buginese people of Indonesia.

- **Mahu (Māhū), Hawaii:** People who exhibit both feminine and masculine traits. In precolonial days, they were highly respected priests, healers, and teachers and are now—after a century of stigmatization—regaining recognition.

- **Sworn virgins (burrnesha), Albania:** Women who take vows of celibacy and live as men, often as a way to avoid arranged marriages.

- **Mino or Dahomey Amazons, Benin:** Known as female warriors, the Mino were a fierce army of women. While they would be considered gender non-conforming from a Western lens, it's unclear if the group considered themselves as a separate, non-binary gender or a religious/specialized subset (there's a lot of debate among historians).

- **Sekrata, Madagascar:** People in the Antandroy and Hova groups who are AMAB but raised from a young age as women. They are considered sacred and believed to carry spiritual powers.

- **Sistergirls and Brotherboys, Tiwi Islands, Australia:** Transgender people of the Aboriginal community.

- **Travesti, much of South America:** People AMAB who identify with various or all aspects of feminine gender expression.

Here's a deeper dive into some of the many groups who identify outside of the binary.

TWO-SPIRITS OF THE UNITED STATES AND CANADA

In many North American Indigenous tribes, there is a concept of a third gender, now often referred to as *two-spirit* people. The role these individuals played varied widely according to each community's language, spirituality, and established gender roles. Some believe two-spirits are able to see the world through the eyes of both genders, acting as forces of balance between feminine and masculine energies. Note that two-spirit does not indicate the sexual or romantic orientation of an individual, only their gender.

»WE'WHA, A ZUNI LHAMANA (TWO-SPIRIT)

SARIMBAVY OF MADAGASCAR

Gender-non-conforming individuals in colonial Madagascar are referred to as Sarimbavy. Boys who exhibit more interest in traditionally feminine tasks, fashion, or social interactions are raised wearing women's clothing and work in feminine roles. Within their communities, Sarimbavy are highly respected, participating in sacred events as spiritual conduits imbued with supernatural powers. The Sarimbavy were described by early 1900s colonialist research, specifically a text published in 1933 by German psychiatrist Iwan Bolch, *Anthropological Studies on the Strange Sexual Practices of All Races and All Ages*.

PHUYING, PHUYING PRAPHET SONG, AND KATHOEYS OF THAILAND

Phuying ("women"), phuying praphet song ("second kind of woman"), and kathoeys are people assigned male at birth but who live as women. Kathoeys are legally recognized as a third gender, though most non-cis people do not identify with that term. Thailand is outwardly very accepting of these people (partly in an effort to encourage gay tourism), but discrimination, homophobia, and transphobia are still major issues, especially outside of major cities. Homosexuality was decriminalized in the 1950s, but there are few explicit legal rights or protections for LGBTQIA+ people: There are no hate-crime laws, same-sex unions are not legal, and transgender and intersex individuals are often left out of human rights and policy discourse.

ANCIENT INCA OF PERU

Third-gender people (quariwarmi) were shamans who performed rituals in which they accessed the past and present, masculine and feminine, and the living and the dead. These rituals sometimes involved homosexual behavior.

HIJRAS OF INDIA

Hijras are one of the most well-known third-gender populations. Made up of transgender women or intersex people who dress in women's clothing, the hijra occupy a unique role in Indian society. However, not all transgender people in India are hijras. The hijra presence in religious texts dates back thousands of years to the Indian epic poem *Ramayana* (from around 500 BC). The hijra had long been portrayed as holding mystical abilities in Hindu culture, but after colonization their identity became feared and shamed. Hijras face violence, ostracization, and exploitation, and most survive off of sex work. However, India is taking steps to protect and help transgender people by providing gender-affirming medical services and has legally recognized the third gender.

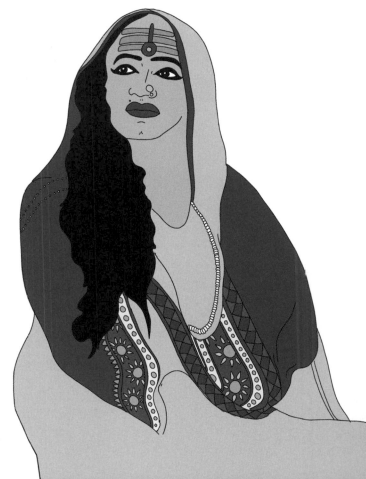

»LAXMI NARAYAN TRIPATHI, A HIJRA WHO BECAME THE FIRST TRANSGENDER PERSON TO REPRESENT ASIA PACIFIC IN THE UN IN 2008

Shakespeare

In fourteenth-century Elizabethan England, women were prohibited from acting on stage. Therefore, in Shakespeare's plays, boys and men (usually younger actors whose voices had not yet deepened) were cast in female roles. Gender bending was nodded to in many of his plays, which added richness and humor to the characters, and rebelled against the gender rules of the times.

Cuttlefish

Cuttlefish are some of the most masterful camouflagers in the animal kingdom. Since males outnumber females four to one, and females are picky (turning down 70 percent of "offers"), competition is fierce during mating season. Large males attempt to gain the attention of females through posturing or displays of flashy skin patterning. But don't count out smaller males: One of their tricks is to change their patterning and color to mimic that of females, sometimes even pretending to carry an egg sac. Then while two large males are fighting it out, the sneaky smaller male slips past them unnoticed and mates with the females. Some cuttlefish have even been spotted with half-and-half skin markings—a male pattern that faces the female cuttlefish next to them and a female pattern that faces males.

Brains win over brawn.

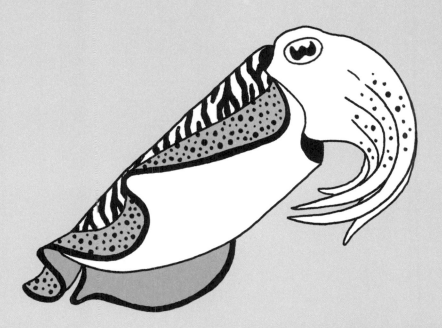

Spotlight on:
Frida Kahlo (1907–1954)

"I used to think I was the strangest person in the world but then I thought, there are so many people in the world, there must be someone just like me who feels bizarre and flawed in the same ways I do. I would imagine her and imagine that she must be out there thinking of me too. Well, I hope that if you are out there and read this and know that, yes, it's true. I'm here, and I'm just as strange as you."

—FRIDA KAHLO

Frida Kahlo was a revolutionary in many senses. She existed in the in-betweens: between gender, sexuality, and race. She was engaged in a lifelong exploration of inconsistent realities within herself and in the world around her.

Kahlo contracted polio at age six (which caused a lifelong limp), and twelve years later she was involved in a serious bus accident that left her bedridden for several months and permanently disabled. While bedridden, she delved into painting self-portraits, saying, "I paint myself because I am often alone, and I am the subject I know best." Her gender fluidity was unabashedly represented in her work, as were miscarriage, heteronormativity, birth, and disability, topics still not fully accepted into non-taboo dialogue.

Self-identified as mestizo (mixed race) and bisexual, Kahlo explored her existence outside of normative societal categories through fashion and painting.

Kahlo had an iconic and recognizable look: striking black hair, a beautiful face with an intense stare, a dark mustache, and of course, her famous unibrow. Her sartorial style spanned a wide spectrum, from men's suits to ornate traditional Mexican dresses.

Her unconventional and often toxic marriage to painter Diego Rivera was marked by affairs on both sides, Kahlo's with both men and women—Communist Leon Trotsky, famous women such as Josephine Baker, and even some of Diego's own mistresses.

Not only did she live outside of societal restrictions, but both her work and personal story continue to push others to confront the in-betweens.

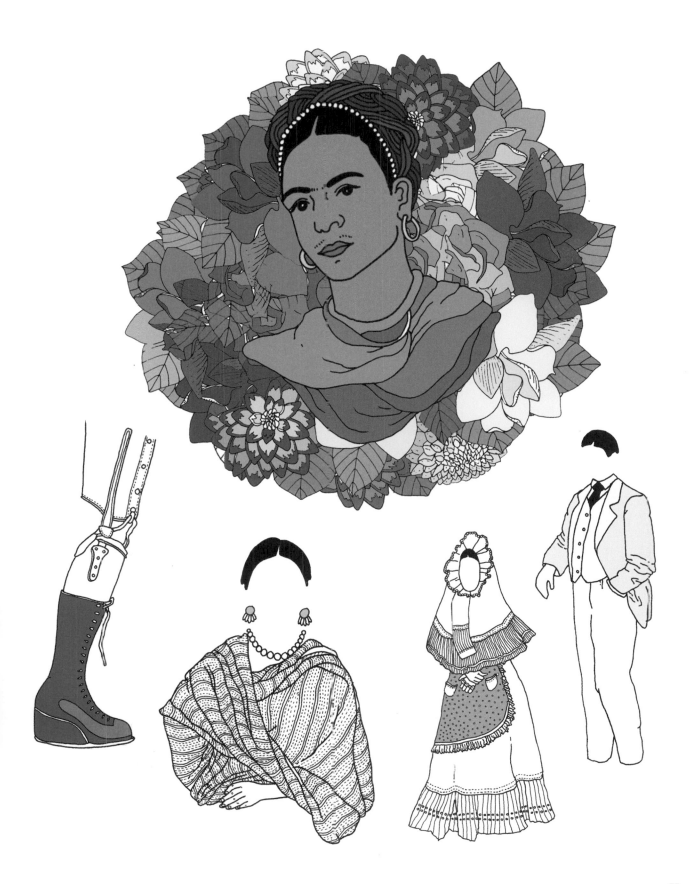

Biology Doesn't Make Gender

There is a debate in the scientific and social world about how much of a factor biology plays in the difference between men, women, and everyone in between and beyond. There are theories and findings that are completely contradictory to one another:

- That men and women have entirely different ways of processing info, problem solving, and experiencing emotions, and that they have areas of inherent intelligence based on their biology

- That genders and sexes are not tied to biological factors in any way

- That biology and social constructs weave together to create our individual and collective gender identities

"The human brain may be a mosaic, but it is one with predictable patterns."

–"PATTERNS IN THE HUMAN BRAIN MOSAIC DISCRIMINATE MALES FROM FEMALES," BY ADAM M. CHEKROUD, EMILY J. WARD, MONICA D. ROSENBERG, AND AVRAM J. HOLMES

Much of the scientific debate revolves around how our brains influence our behavior. As discussed in the physical sex section of this book, anatomy and gender can be intricately tied, but anatomical and biological sex do not determine the gender of a person.

Neuroscience gets hazier. Many scientific publications have findings with an anti-transgender bias, viewing biology as "immutable and factual." This leads to gender essentialism, the belief that there are two fundamentally different categories of humans: men and women, each of which share a baseline set of characteristics (their "essence") determined by their biological makeup. Studies have shown that asking people to read scientific articles favoring gender essentialism (whether they are factual or not) increases prejudice.

There is evidence that all brains have a mixed bag of male and female characteristics that are heavily influenced by the gender in which you were raised. This school of thought believes our brains are on a spectrum, very few people (0 to 8 percent) exhibit only masculine or feminine attributes, and the rest have either a mosaic of both extremes or a mix of everything in the middle. How we are raised undoubtedly plays a role in the adults we become, even if our genders would most likely turn out the same no matter what our upbringing is. Trauma, parenting style, and role models certainly influence how we think of and present ourselves.

"In humans, the fact that you're raised as a particular gender from the instant that you're born of itself exerts a biological impact on your brain."

–NEUROSCIENTIST MARGARET M. MCCARTHY

Sex is an important and necessary thing to take into account in many medical and biological contexts including development of drug treatments, mental illness treatments, and reproductive health. However, the need to categorize our brain functions into two distinctive and deterministic categories is not a useful way of assessing how we will all behave or what we will be skilled at.

"Talking about average differences is misleading if that's all we do. The brain is not a uniform entity that behaves as something male or something female, and it doesn't behave the same way in all contexts."

–ANNE FAUSTO-STERLING, PROFESSOR EMERITA OF BIOLOGY AND GENDER DEVELOPMENT AT BROWN UNIVERSITY

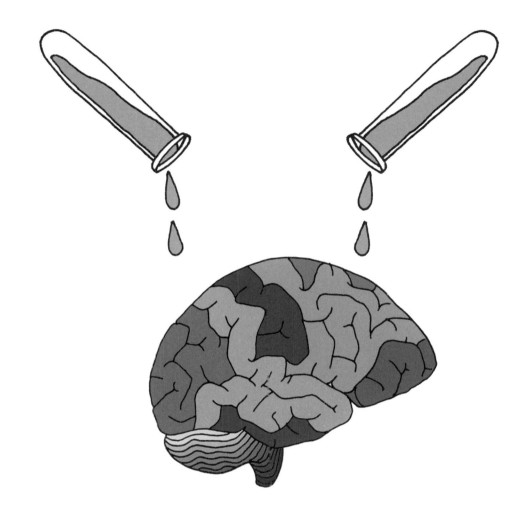

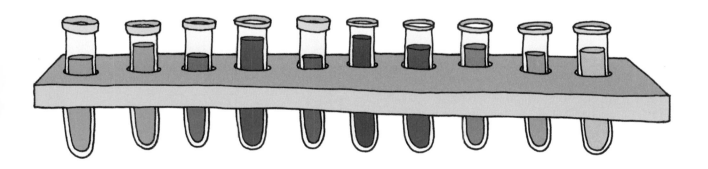

The Brain Weight Myth

In the 1800s, it was a commonly held scientific theory that men were more intelligent than women because their brains were larger, and that white people were more intelligent than all other races for the same reason.

Paul Broca was the man behind the theory that "proved" these biological differences. He obtained data from a comparative study of the craniums of cadavers but skewed the data with his own racism and sexism. Unfortunately, he put forward his data as objective fact and indisputable science before there were standards for medical studies.

Broca wrote, "We might ask if the small size of the female brain depends exclusively upon the small size of her body. Tiedemann [German anatomist] has proposed this explanation. But we must not forget that women are, on the average, a little less intelligent than men, a difference which we should not exaggerate but which is, nonetheless, real. We are therefore permitted to suppose that the relatively small size of the female brain depends in part upon her physical inferiority and in part upon her intellectual inferiority."

He has, of course, been proven completely wrong. Let me repeat: **This is not scientific data.** There are no intellectual disparities between races, and there are no intellectual disparities between men and women; but Broca's theory, which was bolstered by "science," has been influential for two centuries.

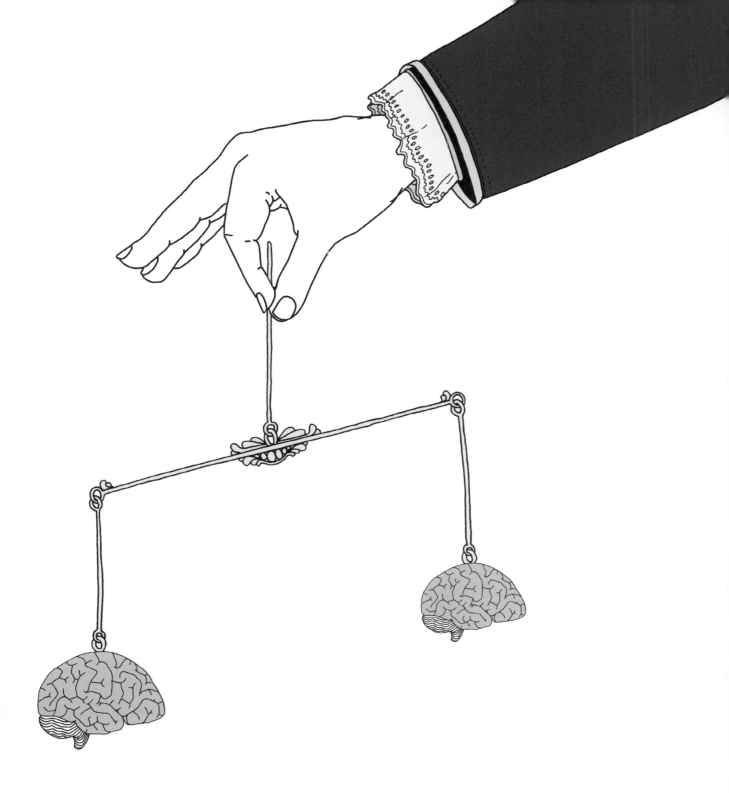

Women in STEM

There are immense systemic obstacles that prevent girls from having equal educational and work opportunities, particularly in STEM fields (science, technology, engineering, and math). White men have dominated STEM fields, both historically and currently. In fact, women, and especially women of color, do not have access to STEM resources in schools and are often discouraged from studying these subjects due to expected gender roles that are reinforced in childhood.

There is an assumption that children assigned female at birth (AFAB) will not be interested in STEM careers down the line, and therefore, parents often do not encourage early exploration of these ideas. This leaves girls with less confidence in those skills than their male counterparts. "It's possible that in the long run, the stereotypes will push young women away from the jobs that are perceived as requiring brilliance, like being a scientist or an engineer," says Lin Bian, researcher of developmental psychology at Stanford. There are super simple ways of engaging that are often reserved for boys' play, like using simple engineering, building toys, digging up insects to inspect, or looking at books about outer space.

Lack of role models is also an issue. "Schools that serve minority and lower-income neighborhoods tend to employ teachers with fewer years of experience and less specialized training in math and science than schools in white and upper-income neighborhoods," according to a 2012 National Science Foundation report. Although there are programs that increase opportunities for women, and women are progressively occupying more space in STEM fields, there is still a lot of ground to cover to reach equal representation.

So if you're a parent, learn alongside your children and experience the world through their curiosity. Girls are no less interested in or capable of excelling in STEM fields—we just need to create a system that reinforces that.

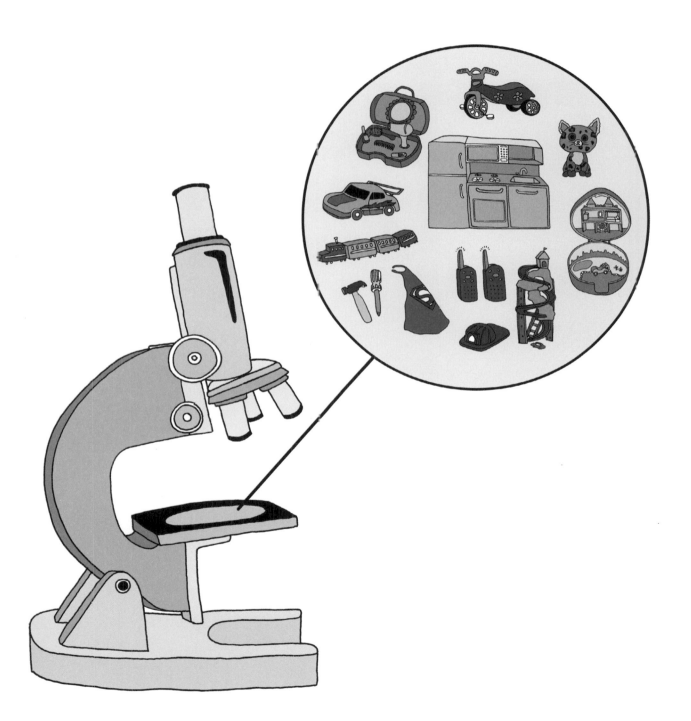

1800s Clothing

Gendered clothing for young children was not a culturally normalized concept in the United States until the early twentieth century. Before then, for centuries, young children under the age of six or seven wore white dresses, which were popular for their practicality—easy to bleach and easy to pass down to child after child. Boys switched to pants and shirts around the time when they received their first haircut at age seven.

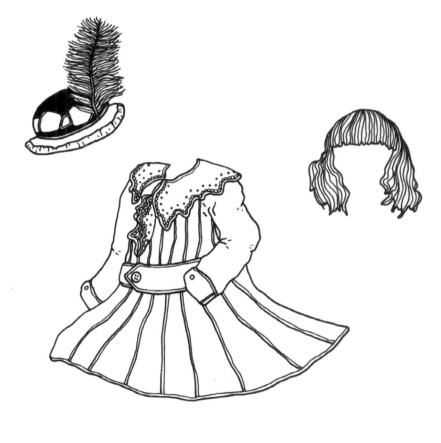

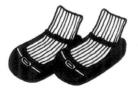

≈OUTFIT OF FRANKLIN D. ROOSEVELT, 1884

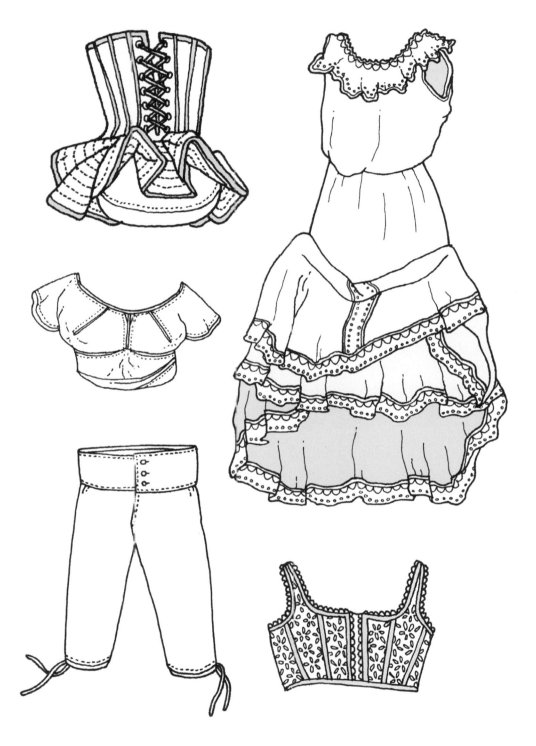

WOMEN'S UNDERWEAR OF THE 1800s WAS DEFINITELY NOT DESIGNED FOR COMFORT

Louis XIV and the High Heel

This outfit could be in a modern-day drag show.

After the death of his father, Louis XIV was made the king of France and ruled for seventy-two years, beginning at the age of four (obviously the age at which you become fit to make national decisions).

While we might see this fashion as being emasculating or effeminate with its lace, high heels, and long fur jacket (not to mention Louis's long hair), at the time it was an outfit that unequivocally represented the wealth, power, and masculinity of a king. Unlike today, where fashion is different per gender, in France in the 1700s, fashion demonstrated a demarcation between social classes. There was gendered clothing, but only upper-class nobility (of both genders) wore specific kinds of garments, fabrics, and aesthetics.

In this period, practicality (or lack thereof) was the indicator of wealth. Louis XIV made high heels popular worldwide, not for women, but for men. He was relatively short (5'4") and heels boosted his physical stature of power. The high heel represented a lack of practicality: the higher the heel, the less easily one could do manual labor—the work of the lower class in French society. The height of the heel indicated the wealth of the wearer. High heels were banned for anyone outside of the royal court, though knockoffs were worn by people who knew the king would never be looking down to notice their feet (and catch them).

Women of upper-class status began wearing heeled shoes to masculinize their fashion, to indicate wealth and proximity to power. Heel styles diverged over the course of the 1700s, with chunkier, more square shapes for men's shoes and more slender, tapered shoes for women.

It wasn't until the 1800s—the Age of Enlightenment—when practicality returned to favor in upper-class society. Men's fashion moved away from ornate luxury, starting a more pronounced gender division in Western European fashion. When the intellectual Enlightenment era took hold, men were expected to pursue academic, practical, and artistic endeavors. In contrast, women were expected to be submissive, emotional, and remain uneducated, all of which was accentuated by the impractical nature of the heel, which became solely associated with femininity.

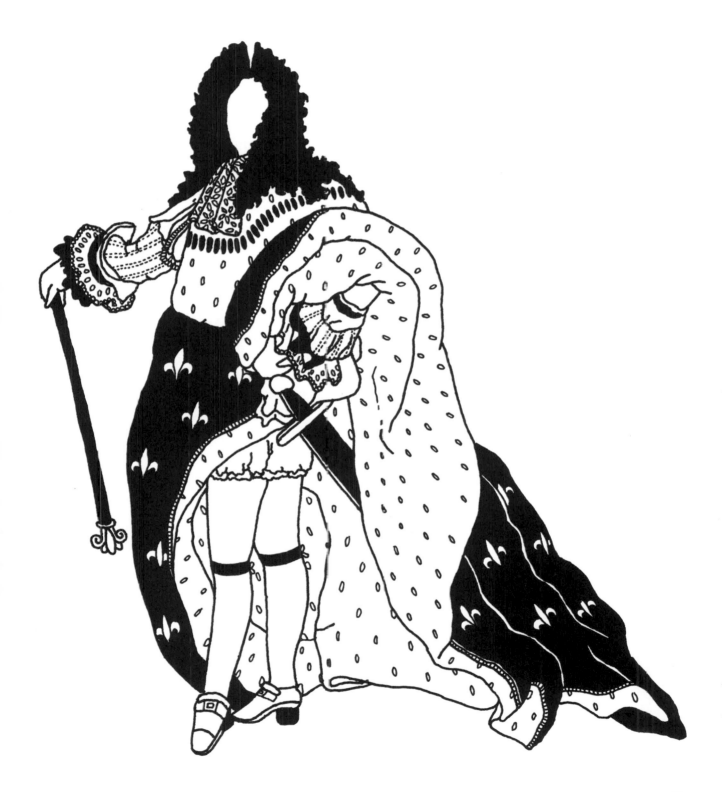

Spotlight on:

Coco Chanel (1883–1971)

Pants: We all wear 'em. But we didn't before Coco Chanel.

The French clothing designer Coco Chanel brought women into the modern era by incorporating elements of menswear into everyone's wear. After World War I, Chanel introduced a radical idea: design affordable clothing for women as a fashionable symbol of liberation from constrictive corsets.

In 1926, Chanel released her version of the little black dress, and *Vogue* dubbed it "Chanel's Ford." Just like the Model T brought the automobile to the everyman, her dress was accessible to women of all classes.

After World War II, when fabrics were expensive, Chanel embraced this constraint, building her fashion brand on unconventional practicality. Black was elevated beyond the realm of funerals, costume jewelry was paired with simpler clothing as a cheaper way to maintain femininity, and suits invoked the power of men for women entering the post-war workplace. Although scandalous at the time, pants were introduced as women's wear, which provided more comfort and practicality for women.

Chanel changed the world of fashion in liberating ways for women; however, behind the scenes, Chanel was involved romantically and financially with the Nazi party and may have served as a member of the Nazi military intelligence. Many of the details are well documented surrounding her partnership with a German officer and her business dealings that were influenced by anti-Semitism. Her legacy in fashion is much more well known, but it's still important to be aware of the darker sides of those we admire.

The staples of today's women's fashion—comfortable fabrics, simple silhouettes, branded perfume, costume jewelry, the little black dress—were all Chanel's creations. While Chanel remains a legacy in the world of fashion, she didn't totally favor the way she shaped women's wear, saying at age eighty-six, "I came up with [trousers] by modesty. From this usage to it becoming a fashion, having 70 percent of women wearing [them] at evening dinner is quite sad."

In my opinion, 70 percent of women wearing trousers to dinner is not sad at all. Not having the option to wear them to dinner is much sadder.

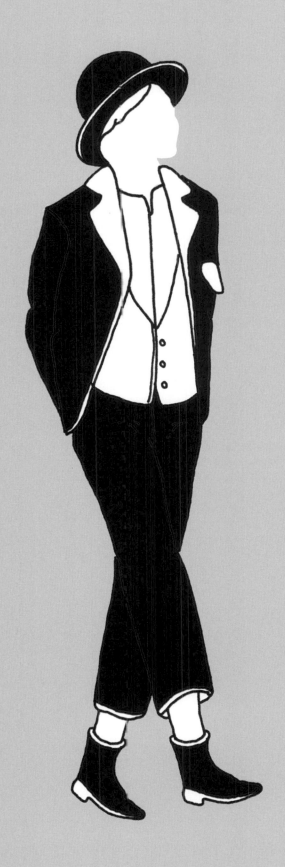

Pink Is for Boys, Blue Is for Girls

World War II was a turning point in color history. Up until then, pink was a unisex color with a slight bent towards masculinity. Pink derives from red, which represents blood, war, and strength. Blue (usually lighter blue) was a girl's clothing color evoking gentleness, daintiness, and passivity. The Western shift in gendered perception of the color pink was largely due to the Nazi's use of the pink triangle on prisoner uniforms to signify gay men, much like yellow stars signified Jews. In 1934, the Gestapo began keeping "pink lists," a record of who was gay and therefore a target of violence or murder. Today the pink triangle has been reclaimed by gay populations as a reminder of the suffering of those persecuted under Nazi rule and in the '80s became a symbol for the fight against the AIDS epidemic.

An article in the June 1918 issue of the trade publication *Earnshaw's Infants' Department* stated, "The generally accepted rule is pink for the boys, and blue for the girls. The reason is that pink, being a more decided and stronger color, is more suitable for the boy, while blue, which is more delicate and dainty, is prettier for the girl." After the war, men returned to reclaim their positions as workers and businessmen, adopting blue as a power color. Women were pushed out of the workplace and back into the home, taking pink with them.

Starting from a very young age, children are given toys and clothing that prep them to fulfill traditional gender roles. Girls are given crowns and pink clothing in everything from dresses to bikinis. They get makeup kits, dolls, toy kitchens, and malls inundating them with messages about motherhood, beauty standards, and domesticity. Meanwhile, boys are given blue clothing adorned with trucks, planes, and dinosaurs, and they play with cars, guns, building blocks, trains, and plastic tools. They're taught to value practical labor, engineering, figuring out how things work, and, sadly, violence.

Childhood interaction with gendered objects, imagination games, and gender roles during play (for example, playing house vs. playing cops and robbers) has a profound impact on self-perception and gender expectation. Children engage in play that mimics the roles they see in the adults around them and are influenced by marketing strategies that enforce gender norms.

Boys are taught to steer away from pink but have no natural aversion to it. Girls are taught to value themselves by beauty standards but have no genetic aversion to dirt. By letting kids determine what they naturally like rather than suggesting what they should like, we will produce a generation of kids who are able to navigate the complicated world of gender with more confidence, skills, and sensitivity to equity.

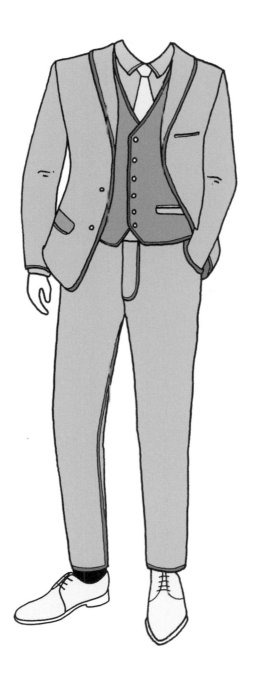

Accessing femininity within oneself and being emotional, vulnerable, and affectionate doesn't make men less male.

Power doesn't equal strength.

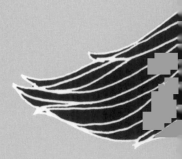

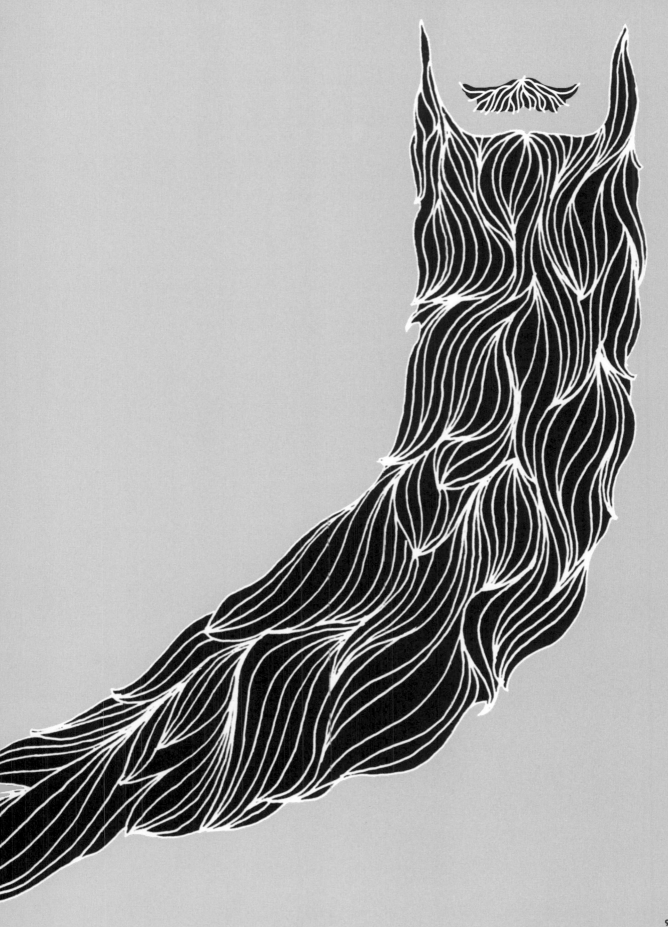

Boys Will Be Boys

How Toxic Masculinity Shapes the Male Population

The term *toxic masculinity* has reentered the public sphere following the waves of sexual harassment incidents coming to light on the national stage. Toxic masculinity describes a dynamic in which men express their gender identity by suppressing emotions, expressing feelings with anger rather than vulnerability, and exhibiting dominance over one another and women/other genders. This societal idea of how to achieve masculinity leads to toxic behaviors such as sexual harassment, domestic and sexual violence, misogyny, homophobia, and substance abuse. **Let's be clear: toxic masculinity is different from masculinity.** When masculinity is expressed in harmful and negative ways, it becomes toxic masculinity. However, that does not mean that all men who exhibit masculine behaviors are engaging in toxic masculinity.

The term has a surprising origin in the mythopoetic men's movement of the 1990s. This movement claimed that men were stripped of some fundamental masculinity during the Industrial Revolution and there was a need to restore a sense of the "deep masculine." According to this group, men's loss of masculinity was the direct result of spending excessive time around women, being falsely (in their minds) accused by feminists of sexism, no longer having noncompetitive male bonding time, and stifled emotional expression. It's deeply ironic that toxic masculinity originally pertained to society's (perceived) toxic effects upon men, versus the toxic effects men's behavior has on women and other genders.

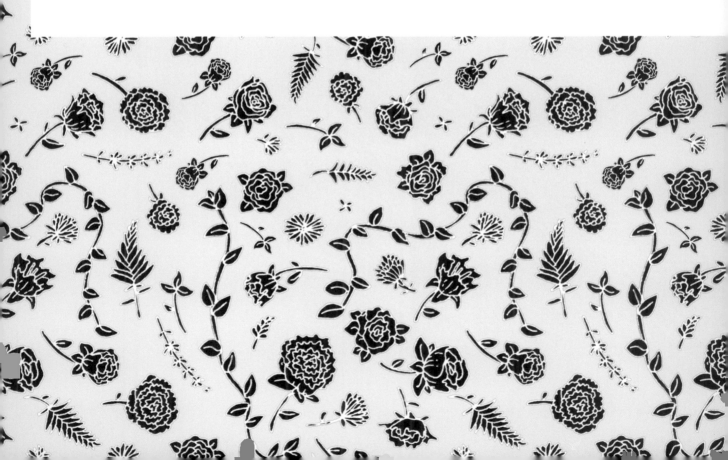

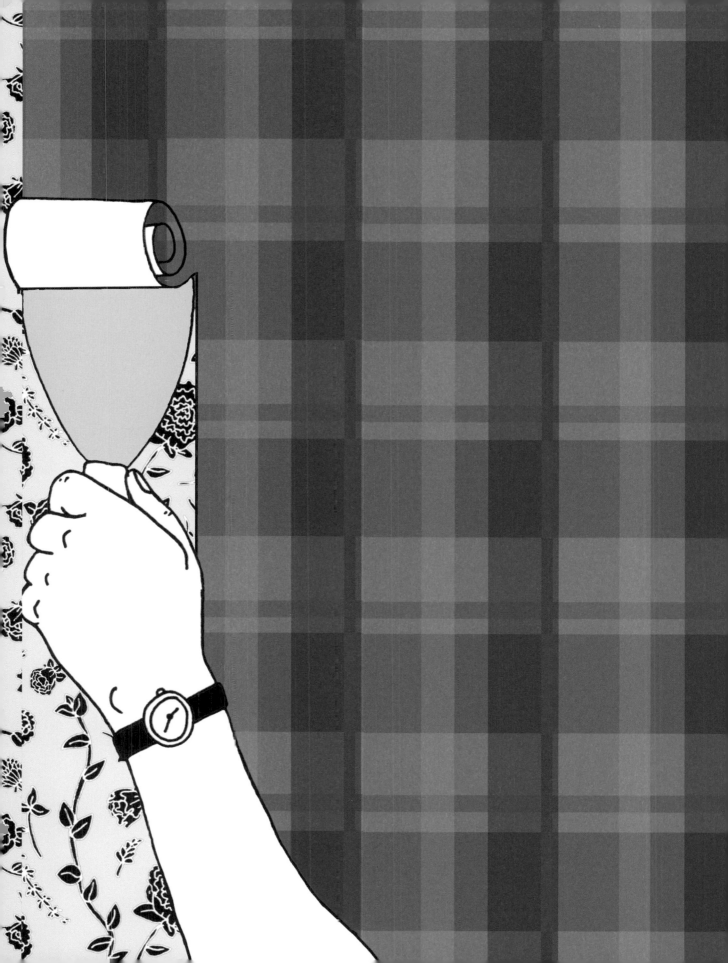

Spotlight on:

Anohni

"Everyone has a spectrum of masculinity and femininity inside them. In every individual, a war of misogyny is raging. Every man is repressing and oppressing the femininity within themselves, raising up male values as governing values. Because that's what we've been taught to do, just as every woman has. Misogyny isn't just something that affects women. It affects men."

—ANOHNI

Anohni, formerly known as Antony Hegarty of Antony and the Johnsons (named in honor of Marsha P. Johnson), is a transgender singer and musician known for her genre-bending music and outspoken stance on gender, environmentalism, and the connection between the two.

There is so much tied to fame and identity, so much pressure to remain in the identity that people know and praise. The process of changing one's personal and public gender identity is brave and incredible, particularly when one's name is how they are known by the world. Anohni had had an almost twenty-year career with Antony and the Johnsons. She released her first album under the name Anohni in 2015. It was a new professional identity, though it had been a name used in her personal life for quite some time. She stated, "To call a person by their chosen gender is to honor their spirit, their life and contribution."

Like it or not, we take cues from famous people— what to expect of ourselves and others, and what is culturally accepted. To see Anohni shift identities is important. She's a shining example that one's identity should not be hidden because of fame. And in fact, her ability to change and morph her identity while in the public spotlight gives visibility to the fact that identity does grow.

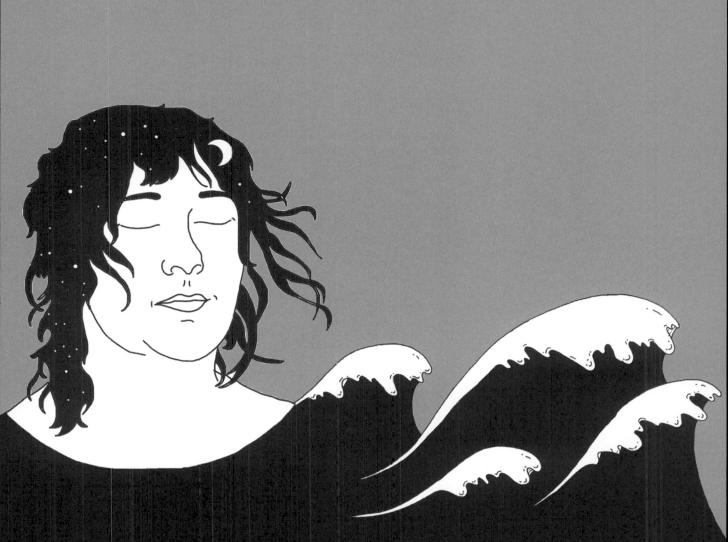

The Patriarchy

Patriarchy is defined by *Merriam-Webster* as the "social organization marked by the supremacy of the father in the clan or family, the legal dependence of wives and children, and the reckoning of descent and inheritance in the male line." Today, the word is commonly used to describe a society or system of governance in which men (particularly straight white men) occupy the highest tier in a power structure, hold most (if not all) of the power, and oppress those who are not straight white men. A patriarchy's influence manifests in more abstract, subtle ways than simply a CEO or president having physical power over a company or country.

We experience patriarchy in micro and macro ways.

MICRO:

- You probably have your dad's last name.
- If you marry a man, you might take his last name.
- Men generally do less childcare at home.
- Your male coworker speaks over you.

MACRO:

- Most world leaders have historically been men, and as of 2018, only three countries have majority-women parliaments.
- Sex-selective abortions (particularly during China's one-child policy) were/are done in order to choose male children over female children.
- Women make less money than men (an average of 82 cents to the dollar that white men make). The breakdown of women's pay discrepancy in the United States varies significantly depending on race and ethnicity. Asian women make 90 cents to the dollar, white women make 79 cents to the dollar, Black women make 62 cents to the dollar, Native American women make 57 cents to the dollar, and Latinas make 54 cents to the dollar.
- The legality of abortion is decided by the government (ahem, men).
- Most history is and has been written by men. *His*-story.

On the surface it would seem that only women suffer under the patriarchy. And while they certainly suffer much more than men do (ever been told to "smile more"? That's the patriarchy asking), the patriarchy affects everyone and causes a dangerous cycle of oppression. A patriarchal society requires men to embody all of the traits associated with masculinity: aggressiveness, dominance, and strength. Men must hold power to be men, thus continuing the cycle of gendered oppression. Ironically, this cycle does not serve men well. Patriarchy enforces a rigid gender divide in which there is only one way to be a boy who will grow up to be one kind of man. It shames young boys for things like wearing pink, crying, and not liking sports. Men raised in a rigid patriarchy will almost certainly be exposed to and/or perpetuate toxic masculinity to some degree.

While it materially serves men to be in power, it sets them up for emotional failure. In any oppressive dynamic, it's not the job of the oppressed (in this case, women or non-cis men) to teach their oppressors how to be less oppressive. Yet, because marginalized people have the most informed perspective on the ill effects of the patriarchy (through experience), they're the ones burdened with challenging these forces. Women, viewed as the "emotional gender," do that work constantly for men in the form of emotional labor: using emotional energy to manage their own feelings and those around them, which can be exhausting. It happens at home in the form of childcare, managing extended family obligations, and initiating dialogues about relationship issues. This work is generally not acknowledged, appreciated, or compensated. Most jobs traditionally held by women are jobs based on emotional labor: nurses, service workers, social workers/therapists, daycare workers, and teachers. However, emotional labor demands occur at any workplace where women are expected to do the work of maintaining relationships or "keeping the ship afloat."

This system of male dominance that has persisted for thousands of years must shift to make society more equitable. Here are some ways that men can do their part to fight patriarchy:

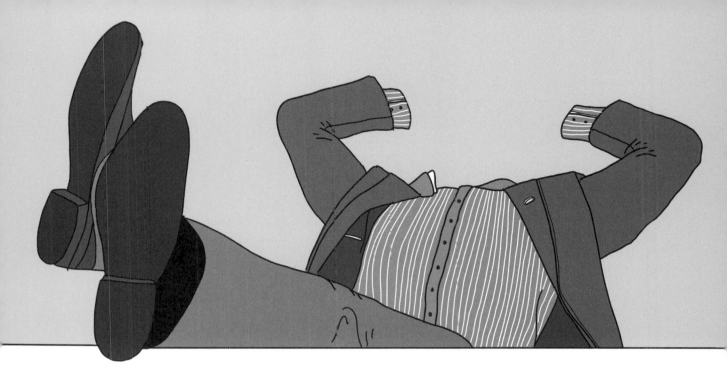

1. **Admit you're part of the problem, even if you're not doing anything intentionally.** Admit that you have privilege, even if you don't feel you benefit directly from it. We do not choose our privileges, but we must acknowledge them before we're able to understand our impact on others.

2. **Listen to women, trans people, genderqueer people, and children.** Your opinions are not inherently more intelligent, more original, or more important than anyone else's—you've just been given a louder megaphone and a bigger audience. Practice listening more than talking when in a group. Notice if you are interrupting, and if you are, notice whom you are interrupting.

3. **Teach your children that it is not only acceptable, but also good and healthy, to be emotional.** Things are sad and hard as a kid sometimes — it's okay to cry about them! Teach them that gender is a broad spectrum of possibility and there is no singular way to express it. Treat your children like they're important, smart people who have ideas worth listening to.

4. **Go to therapy to learn how to better access your emotions and take on your fair share of emotional labor.** If you don't have access to therapy, talk to your male friends about how to do better before asking your friends who are not men. Remember, those you oppress should not have to teach you to be less oppressive.

5. **Challenge your male friends, family, or coworkers when they're being sexist, racist, homophobic, ableist, or ageist.** It can be uncomfortable and scary to call out the person making offensive remarks, but it's incredibly important to hold yourself and your community accountable for oppressive or harmful behavior.

6. **Do not tolerate discussions, insinuations, or allusions to sexual harassment** or "locker room talk" about violence by those you know. *For real.*

7. **Acknowledge the pay disparity by donating part of your paycheck** to an organization that supports a cause that serves women, queer people, trans people, rape crisis centers, domestic violence shelters, STEM programs for girls, and small, local fundraisers for people in need.

8. **Show up for women.** Attend rallies, volunteer for events, and donate your time, your skills, and your position of power to boost the messages of those around you who don't have access to the same audience.

9. **Think about the way that intersectionality plays a role in the patriarchy.** So, you've got a job, right? Are you white? Did you get the job over someone of color? Would you be willing to offer it to a woman or POC man or queer person as equally qualified as you? How about making sure your boss pays them as well as he would you? How does your race affect your position within the patriarchy? How about your class? Your sexuality?

10. **Educate yourself.** See the resources list (page 196) for suggestions.

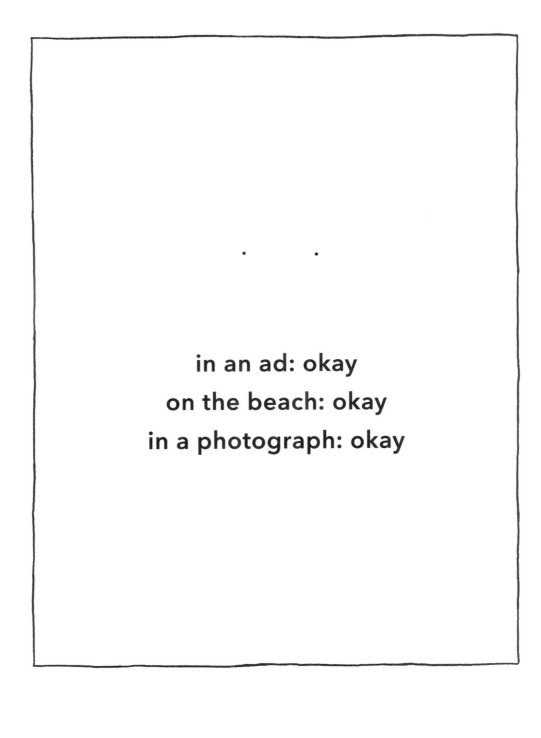

in an ad: okay
on the beach: okay
in a photograph: okay

in an ad: not okay

on the beach: not okay

in a photograph: not okay

Lions

In the Mombo area of the Moremi Game Reserve of Botswana's Okavango Delta, there are lionesses who have manes and occasionally engage in male mating behavior. This is most likely due to a genetic trait within the area's population that results in increased testosterone. This theory is borne out by the fact that the maned lionesses seem infertile (they are seen mating but never get pregnant).

These lionesses often trick outsiders, protecting the pride from predators and competitors.

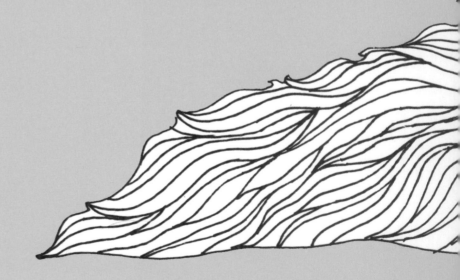

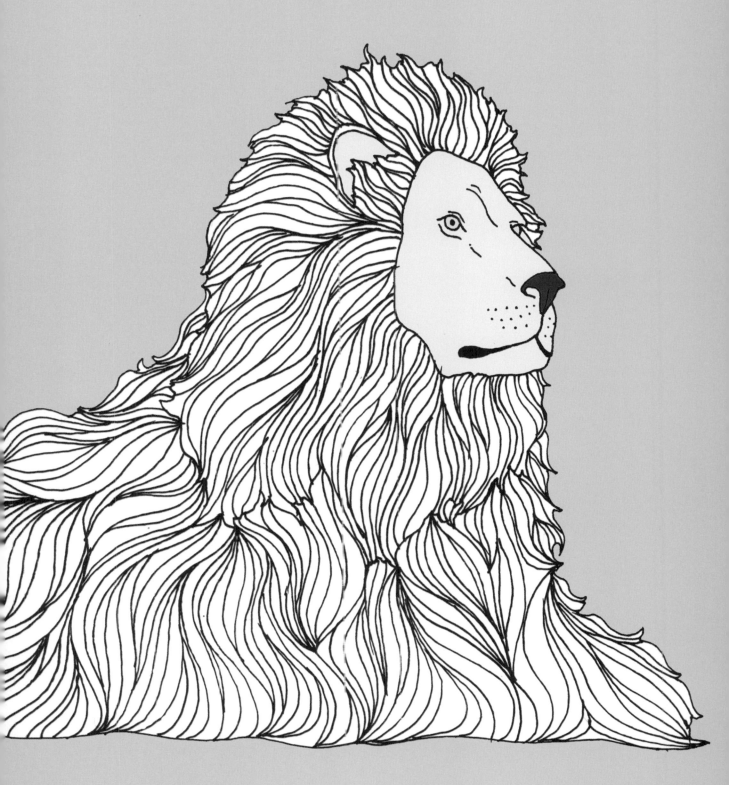

Sports

Sports have had a long history of discrimination against people for their race, gender, or both. While sports have become more integrated and genders are better represented, there are still some huge leaps to be made to get to a place of equity among those in the world of sports (or who would like to be).

One huge problem for athletes—generally those who identify as women—has been that of *sex verification*, a process in which athletes' bodies and anatomy, chromosomes, and hormones are examined to prove that they are a member of the sex for which they are competing.

Sex verification became standardized for the International Association of Athletics Federation (IAAF) in 1950, with the International Olympic Committee (IOC) following in 1968. The first iteration of this testing came in the form of a *nude parade*, which is exactly what it sounds like: female athletes had to show themselves nude to doctors to prove no male athletes were competing as women to gain an unfair advantage.

The verification process evolved in 1968 to use chromosome testing. As explained in the section of this book about intersex people, chromosomes can vary in ways that don't affect someone's gender identity, external anatomy, secondary sexual characteristics, or presentation. To use a chromosome test as a method to determine someone's gender/sex is not only flawed but deeply invasive, discriminatory, and demeaning.

The IAAF ended official gender verification in 1992 and the IOC banned it in 1999, but incredibly gendered "suspicion-based" testing is still allowed. Transgender athletes were allowed to compete but were required to have obtained official legal documentation, and to have undergone sex reassignment surgery and hormone therapy "appropriate for the assigned sex."

The current form of these tests is hormone testing to determine if a competitor has hyperandrogenism, a condition where testosterone levels are elevated in women. Hyperandrogenism is viewed to give increased athletic performance to those who have it and thus gives them an unfair advantage. Hyperandrogenism does not change someone's gender identity unless they choose that for themselves—it is not to be determined by a doctor or board of an athletic competition. Almost 2 percent of male athletes have testosterone levels in the "typical female range," according to *Scientific American*.

According to the rules of the IOC:

- Men are not tested—at all.
- Transgender men competing in male competitions are not tested.
- Transgender women are required to undergo testing and are allowed to compete in women's sports only if they meet certain testosterone levels.

Some of the athletes affected by these discriminatory practices are:

- **Foekje Dillema** of the Netherlands: Reports vary, some saying she was expelled for refusing testing in 1950 or because of testing results, but the details were never revealed. Either way, gender testing was at the root of her career ending.
- **Ewa Kłobukowska** of Poland: Banned from Olympic competitions and professional sports in 1967 for her XX/XXY chromosomes.
- **Renée Richards** of the United States: A transgender woman who sued the US Tennis Association (and won) after they refused to allow her to play as a woman in the 1976 US Open without undergoing chromosome testing.
- **Maria José Martínez-Patiño** of Spain: Banned from competing in 1986 by the IAAF based on failing her chromosome test. She fought back against that ruling and was later allowed to compete again. Her case raised public awareness of the damage caused by sex verification testing.

- **Pratima Gaonkar** of India: Died by suicide after facing public shame for failing her sex verification test in 2010.

- **Dutee Chand** of India: Banned from the Commonwealth Games in 2014 after she was found to have hyperandrogenism. After taking her case to court, she was granted the right to compete as a female, and as a result the IOC announced it would no longer enforce a qualifying testosterone level for women.

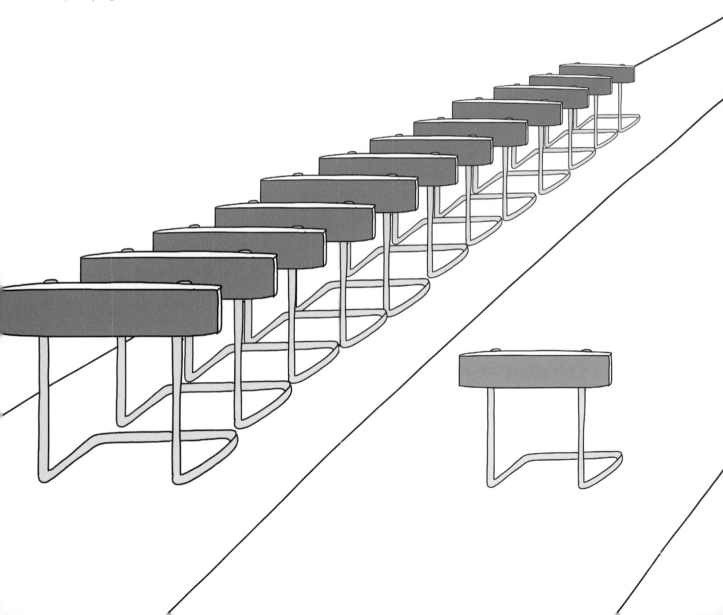

Serena Williams

Intersecting Sports, Race, and Gender

Women, even in professional sports, are expected to have the qualities society has set for women: thinness, femininity, fragility, and nonaggression.

Serena Williams in many ways represents the intersection of sports, race, and gender, and many of the contradictions that identity holds. She has been incredibly successful as a Black woman in a very white sport. Despite her incredible achievements in the sport (she was ranked #1 in the world eight times between 2002 and 2017 by the Women's Tennis Association), she has been frequently judged precisely for what makes her such an incredible athlete—her muscular body (and how she dresses it), her strength, and her assertive take-no-shit attitude. Many of these issues are deeply tied to the subtle and overt ways that Black bodies—particularly women's bodies—are sexualized, objectified, demonized, and criticized in the United States.

In September 2018, Williams was accused of cheating when she received mid-game coaching. She later smashed her racket and was penalized a point. When Williams called the umpire a "thief," he issued a full game penalty, giving her opponent an upper hand. She later received a $17,000 fine for "cheating," "verbal abuse" (of the umpire), and breaking her racket. Men who have tantrums, break their rackets, or yell are rarely penalized for their behavior, and when they are it is not as severe. Shortly after the incident, Williams was depicted in a cartoon as an angry Black woman, with exaggerated racist features—a racist trope that has existed since slavery days and one that is also deeply sexist. She is shown screaming and throwing a tantrum, as indicated by the pacifier on the ground. She defended her behavior, stating, "I'm here fighting for women's rights and for women's equality. . . . For me to say 'thief' and for him to take a game, it made me feel like it was a sexist remark. He's never taken a game from a man because they said 'thief.'"

In 2017, Williams posed nude while pregnant for the cover of *Vanity Fair*. It's an incredible photo full of grace and confidence for which she was praised. Her curves were beautiful when on the cover of a fashion magazine. However, in August 2018, Serena came under fire from the French Tennis Federation's president, Bernard Giudicelli, after she wore a black catsuit (an amazing tight one-piece spandex suit). Giudicelli claimed that "one must respect the game and the place."

Excuse me?

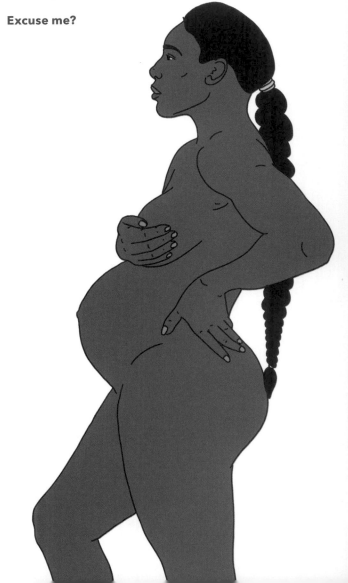

If you've ever watched a professional women's tennis match, you know that the outfits aren't modest. Short skirts with bloomers underneath and tight tank tops are the norm. Williams is known for her outfits on and off the court; they're bold, feminine, and fashion-forward. This catsuit covered her whole body except her arms, so one cannot help but think that the message is not about the clothing itself, but who is wearing it. It implies that Serena's body—a strong, beautiful, Black woman's body that just gave birth one year earlier via C-section—is the offense, not her outfit. This suit was not only fashionable and practical but was medically helpful for Williams. After giving birth, she had problems with blood clots and the snug fit of the tights helps prevent blood clots from forming, allowing her to get back on the court. When asked about the suit, Williams said, "I feel like a warrior in it, a warrior princess . . . from Wakanda, maybe . . . I've always wanted to be a superhero, and it's kind of my way of being a superhero."

The French Tennis Federation is essentially saying, No, we don't want you to feel strong, empowered, healthy, or invincible, we want you to make us more comfortable. Because of her race and gender, people have not only decried Williams's body as masculine, but denied her the respect that she deserves by pinning her successes singularly to her body rather than recognizing her training, dedication, and lifetime of mastering the sport. Yes, her body is her power, but her mastery of the sport is also her power.

In her own words, Williams said, "Oh God, I'll never be a size four! Why would I want to do that, and be that? . . . This is me, and this is my weapon and machine."

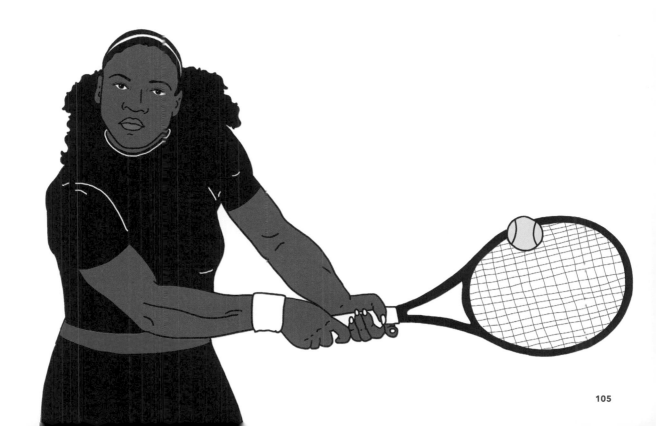

White Feminism

"[In The Feminine Mystique, *Betty Friedan] did not discuss who would be called in to take care of the children and maintain the home if more women like herself were freed from their house labor and given equal access with white men to professions. She did not speak of the needs of women without men, without children, without homes. She ignored the existence of all non-white women and poor white women . . . only women with leisure time and money could actually shape their identities on the model of the feminine mystique."*

—BELL HOOKS, *FEMINIST THEORY: FROM MARGIN TO CENTER*

White feminism is a broad term used to describe feminist movements that focus primarily on issues that affect white women but do not acknowledge white privilege and often actively work against Black women's rights. This is represented in many ways from subtle to overt, small to grand. Second-wave feminism, a movement in the 1960s that came into being in response to women's changing domestic roles in the post-war United States, tends to be a central point of focus when it comes to white feminism's prominence, but white feminism has roots dating back to the suffragist movement and earlier. Susan B. Anthony famously said in 1866, "I will cut off this right arm of mine before I will ever work or demand the ballot for the Negro and not the woman" during a meeting with Frederick Douglass. Her work was as much to get some women the right to vote as it was to keep others from voting at all. Black suffragists like Ida B. Wells and Sojourner Truth worked for women's right to vote and more specifically Black women's right to vote. The fight to give white women equal rights, whether that is voting or a myriad of social and economic advantages, has long been on the agenda to give white women power over Black women.

White writers and thinkers such as Betty Friedan, Gloria Steinem, and Simone de Beauvoir were the public face of the feminist movement, focusing on issues in the workplace, inequality, and sexual freedom while ignoring any semblance of intersectionality around race, class, and sexuality. However, authors and activists such as bell hooks brought with them new voices of POC women who illuminated the struggle of Black women. Black scholars, activists, and thinkers like Florynce Kennedy, Audre Lorde, and bell hooks were often omitted from the conversation, and Black women have been harmed by the whitewashing of large feminist movements.

Today we still praise white women for their feminism far more easily and widely than non-white feminists, despite their consistent failure to include perspectives outside of themselves, their perpetuation of a false sense of gender equity such as the recent transphobic comments made by J. K. Rowling and TERF (trans exclusionary radical feminist) perspectives, or their adoption of outright racist or classist views. While the principles of white feminism do include valuable tenets of equity, they lack complexity and diverse perspectives. Transmisogyny, the discrimination towards trans women stemming from both transphobia and misogyny, is inherently rooted in white feminism, as it ignores and harms the existence of trans identities that historically and currently exist in Indigenous and non-white cultures pre-colonization. The physical characteristics that have been deemed desirable are based on white women's bodies and therefore, the bodies of non-white and trans women are seen as less desirable and less womanly.

We are in a moment of forward momentum, and while white liberal populations revel in being "woke," they're simultaneously ignoring large sectors of the population who began and continue to lead liberation movements. Those who are often in the most marginalized and oppressed groups—Black women and men, Indigenous populations, immigrants, Muslim communities, trans women, disabled folks, sex workers, genderqueer people, and rural populations—are erased as players in the celebration of milestones like gay marriage, the Women's March on Washington, or advancements in AIDS research. *Whitewashing* is when historical events, media representation, and/or credit is given to white people as the face of success, erasing the non-white people who either made it happen or are deserving of praise.

American history as a whole is a one-sided story from the perspective of white men (and later women) and often the women of color who have led socio-political movements haven't been given appropriate credit and recognition for their incredible work. What it boils down to is, **people who face systemic and daily oppression are far more likely to be actively working to dismantle it.** After all, the people who benefit from the oppression of others have no incentive (other than basic decency and a desire for equity) to change the systems that give them power, money, freedom, and control of resources.

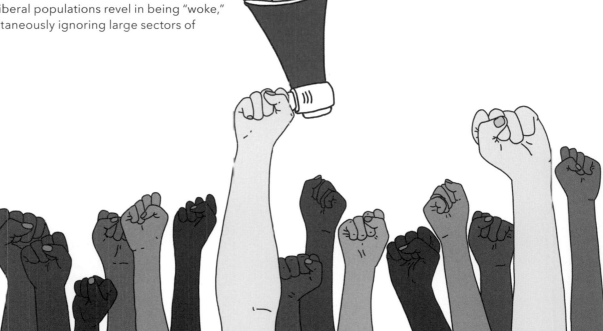

Black Women Are the Backbone of Resistance

These are some of the incredible women who have fought for liberation, rights, and freedom since the 1800s.

Alicia Garza, Patrisse Khan-Cullors, and Opal Tometi, cofounders of Black Lives Matter.

Angela Davis, author, professor, prison abolitionist, cofounder of Critical Resistance.

Assata Shakur, member of the Black Liberation Army.

Audre Lorde, author, librarian, and civil rights activist.

Bessie Coleman, first Black and Native American US pilot.

Claudette Colvin, pioneer of the civil rights movement; arrested for refusing to give up her bus seat nine months before Rosa Parks did.

Coretta Scott King, civil rights activist.

Diane Nash, civil rights activist and a leader and strategist of the student wing of the civil rights movement.

Dr. Dorothy Height, educator and civil rights activist focusing on women's issues in the Black community.

Elaine Brown, former Black Panther chairwoman, prison activist, singer, and writer.

Ella Baker, human and civil rights activist and primary advisor of the Student Nonviolent Coordinating Committee (SNCC).

Fannie Lou Hamer, voting and civil rights activist, vice chairwoman of the Freedom Democratic Party, and cofounder of the National Women's Political Caucus.

Flo Kennedy, lawyer, civil rights activist, and frequent cowboy hat wearer.

Harriet Tubman, abolitionist; escaped slavery and rescued more than three hundred people from slavery in the Underground Railroad.

Ida B. Wells, journalist, suffragist, and cofounder of the National Association for the Advancement of Colored People (NAACP).

Juanita Hall, first African American to win a Tony in 1950 for her role in *South Pacific*.

Katherine Johnson, one of the first Black women mathematicians for NASA.

Kathleen Cleaver, law professor, communications secretary for the Black Panther Party.

Lena Horne, singer, dancer, civil rights activist, actress; the first African American to serve on the Screen Actors Guild board of directors.

Mae Jemison, NASA astronaut, dancer, professor, engineer, physician, and first African American woman to travel in space.

Mahalia Jackson, legendary gospel singer and civil rights activist.

Majora Carter, American urban revitalization strategist and founder of Sustainable South Bronx.

Mary Church Terrell, suffragist, civil rights activist, and one of the first Black women to earn a college degree.

Maya Angelou, poet, singer, civil rights activist, professor, first prominent Black female memoirist, author of *I Know Why the Caged Bird Sings*; awarded three Grammys for spoken word albums, the Presidential Medal of Freedom, and the National Medal of Arts; and earned more than fifty honorary degrees.

Pauli Murray, lawyer, author, priest, and cofounder of the National Organization for Women (NOW).

Phillis Wheatley, first published African American poet.

Rosa Parks, civil rights activist; known as "the mother of the freedom movement" for her refusal to give up her bus seat for a white passenger.

Ruby Bridges, first African American child to desegregate the William Frantz school in New Orleans and founder of the Ruby Bridges Foundation.

Septima Poinsette Clark, educator and civil rights activist, vice president of the Charleston NAACP branch, and founder of Citizenship Schools to teach adults to read in the Deep South.

Shirley Chisholm, first African American to run for the nomination of a major party for president (lost to George McGovern); founding member of the Congressional Black Caucus and Congressional Women's Caucus.

Sojourner Truth, abolitionist, author; helped recruit Black troops to join the Union Army.

And countless others who have and will fight for change.

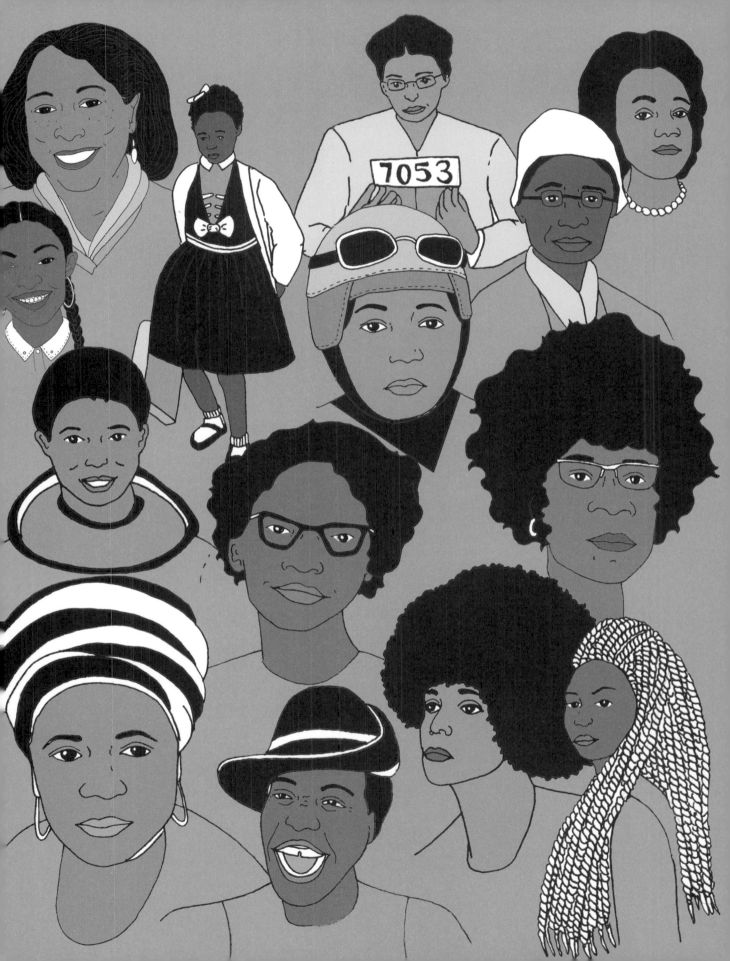

Spotlight on:

Marsha P. Johnson (1945–1992)

Marsha P. Johnson (the P stands for "pay it no mind") was a prominent figure in the LGBTQIA+ liberation movement. Hailed as the "queen of Christopher Street" in New York City, Johnson was a Black transgender woman who performed as a flamboyant drag queen and model and was a lifelong activist. She was deeply beloved by the community she was a part of, but she's often forgotten in the narratives of queer and trans history.

Johnson was on the front lines of the Stonewall Uprising and later became active in the Gay Liberation Front, an activist group fighting to dismantle structural gender inequality and shift the notion that a heteronormative nuclear family was the ideal familial or social centerpoint.

Along with Sylvia Rivera, she founded the STAR (Street Transvestite Action Revolutionaries) house, which provided shelter for homeless queers, young drag queens, sex workers, and transgender youth in New York City. Johnson was a sex worker herself and often homeless, so she knew how important it was to provide services to sex workers in NYC who were often denied adequate services. The program no longer exists, but it became a blueprint for providing services to homeless queer youth.

Into the 1980s, Johnson continued to fight for rights denied to LGBTQIA+ populations and joined ACT UP (AIDS Coalition to Unleash Power). After many incredibly successful direct actions, ACT UP divided into smaller factions and led to organizations that continue to provide some of the largest services to the AIDS community.

Johnson struggled with mental health issues throughout her life, a fact that was used as evidence to support the claim that her 1992 death was a suicide. After she was reported missing, her body was found in the Hudson River. Her community believes Johnson was killed, and in 2012 her friends got NYC police to reopen the case as a possible homicide. Her death remains unsolved, but she continues to be a force of strength, hope, and inspiration, and she's remembered as a leader in the fight for queer liberation. Her legacy as a true queen lives on.

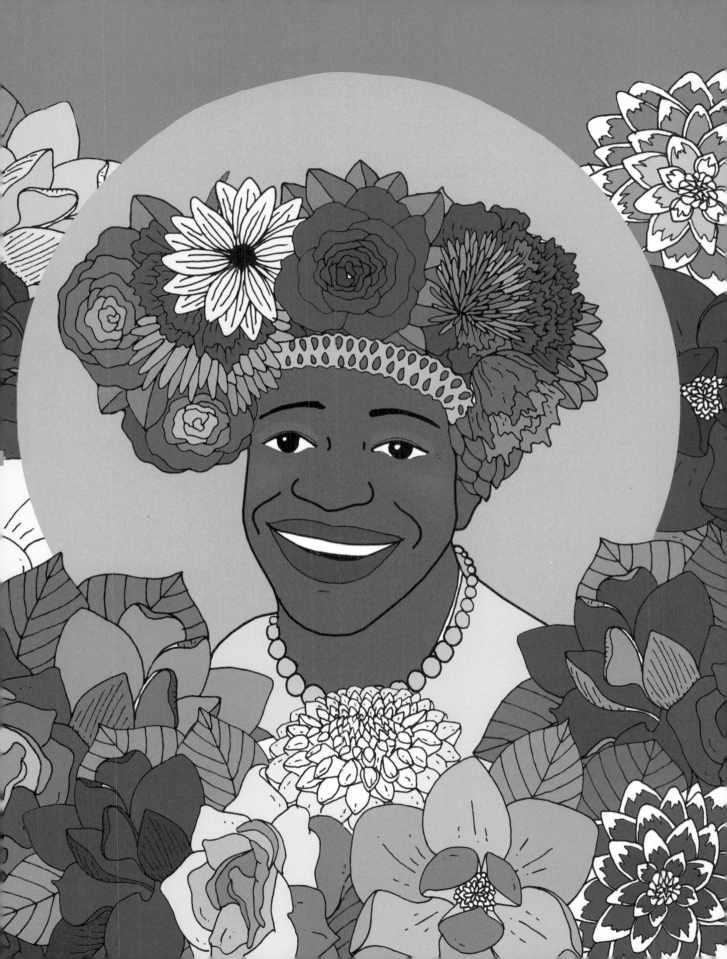

When Black Boys Become Black Men, Part 1

Police Violence Against Black Men

"There can be no keener revelation of a society's soul than the way in which it treats its children."

—NELSON MANDELA

Black boys in the United States are systematically set up to fail.

In order to understand the depth and complexity of most societal problems, we must consider all of our and others' identities. Gender and race are our initial identifying features and when we treat them as the only ones, we fail to recognize crucial points of intersectionality. Race and gender are two major factors behind police violence, school systems failing Black boys, and the judicial system failing Black men.

In the eyes of the police and much of popular culture, Black boys are suspicious in almost any space they occupy—in wealthy white neighborhoods, in Black neighborhoods, and in many public spaces. Since Black males are the most targeted population for unwarranted police stop and frisks (which can be violent or fatal), from childhood on, Black boys are primed to be wary of the police.

Research finds that when police look at an image of two boys, one Black and one white, doing the same thing, they perceive the Black youth as being older than they are and perceive the white youth as being younger.

"Black boys can be misperceived as older than they actually are and prematurely perceived as responsible for their actions during a developmental period where their peers receive the beneficial assumption of childlike innocence."

–"THE ESSENCE OF INNOCENCE: CONSEQUENCES OF DEHUMANIZING BLACK CHILDREN" BY PHILLIP ATIBA GOFF, ET AL.

These misconceptions create a catch-22 for Black youth approached by police, leaving them with few to no safe responses:

- Option 1: Run or resist arrest, and risk being killed.
- Option 2: Follow the officer's instructions, and risk being killed anyway.

The fear of police violence that begins in one's youth is a self-fulfilling prophecy as an adult.

Some of the unarmed Black boys and men killed by police in the past ten years: George Floyd, Sean Reed, Ahmaud Arbery, Ariane McCree, David McAtee, William Green, Tony McDade, Amadou Diallo, Sean Bell, Oscar Grant, Aaron Campbell, Orlando Barlow, Steven Washington, Michael Brown, Freddie Gray, Kendrec McDade, Kimani Gray, Philando Castile, Jordan Edwards, Alton Sterling, Walter Scott, Eric Garner, Tamir Rice. It is also important to mention Trayvon Martin, who was killed by a civilian but is a prominent figure in the conversation about policing and violence toward Black men and boys.

The *Washington Post* found that 234 of the 963 people (24 percent) police shot and killed in 2016 were Black. Only 13.4 percent of the United States' population is Black.

Black people have been 28 percent of those killed by police since 2013 despite being only 13 percent of the population.—MAPPING POLICE VIOLENCE

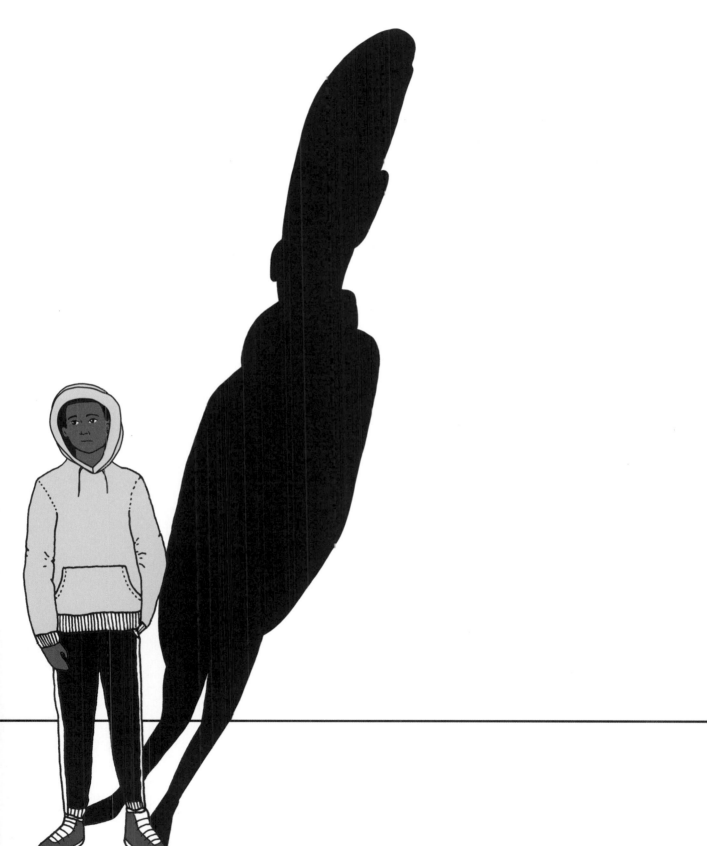

When Black Boys Become Black Men, Part 2

Disproportionate Incarceration of Black Men

The current issue of targeted incarceration of Black men in the United States is not new; it has strong roots in slavery and deeply embedded historical racism.

A quick history lesson will give a huge amount of context to how the systemic racism of the modern-day prison-industrial complex came to be. Before the Civil War, the US government was changing the method of taxation from that of land value to a tax based on population. Since government representation was tied to population, and the larger Northern states had higher populations than the Southern states, Southern states proposed including slaves in population counts to increase their seats in the House. However, they didn't want to pay higher taxes on the increased population, so the Three-Fifths Compromise was reached after much debate. The Three-Fifths Compromise defined slaves as only three-fifths of a white person. It determined that it was acceptable and legal to value a human being as less than a person. This logic increased Southern states' legislative representation, bolstering the political power of slavery states to pass pro-slavery laws.

When slavery was legally abolished in 1865 with the Thirteenth Amendment, it took with it the free labor base in the Southern states, which quickly had economic effects. However, the Thirteenth Amendment contained a loophole that former slaveowners quickly took advantage of: slavery was permissible if it was punishment for a crime. We can see where this leads. Following abolition, "Black Codes" were implemented to define a plethora of "crimes" that could result in incarceration (and thus, available slave labor): vagrancy, interracial relationships, unlawful assembly, or selling produce without permission from an employer. Additionally, orphan minors could be forced into labor.

Convicts were "leased" to the highest bidders to perform manual labor in coal mines, railroads, and logging companies. Sound familiar? During this era, the number of incarcerated people—most of whom were Black men—rose tenfold. This process was as close to slavery as lawmakers could get away with—free labor, race-based violence, and bidding for free labor (paying for people).

While that time seems like the distant past, very little has changed in the ways Black men are treated—the same actions under a different name. The *school-to-prison pipeline* is a term that describes the disproportionate number of underserved Black and brown youth that end up incarcerated, stemming from zero-tolerance policies combined with racially biased punishments in schools. According to the Department of Education, 70 percent of students involved in in-school arrests or referred to law enforcement are Black or Latino. It's important to note that Black and brown boys do not commit more punishable offenses but are punished more frequently and harshly than their white classmates. Because of these policies, most students who experience higher rates of expulsion and suspension are at a higher risk of dropping out and becoming incarcerated.

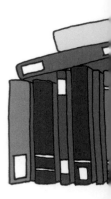

"African-American adults are 5.9 times as likely to be incarcerated than whites and Hispanics are 3.1 times as likely. As of 2001, one of every three Black boys born in that year could expect to go to prison in his lifetime, as could one of every six Latinos—compared to one of every seventeen white boys . . . In 2016, Black Americans comprised 27% of all individuals arrested in the United States—double their share of the total population. Black youth accounted for 15% of all U.S. children yet made up 35% of juvenile arrests in that year."

—REPORT OF THE SENTENCING PROJECT TO THE UNITED NATIONS HUMAN RIGHTS COMMITTEE 2018

Police discriminate against Black men, Black boys, and Black people because of the narrative created by those in power (including the police), which perpetuates systemic oppression. It is crucial to note that modern-day policing descends from slave patrols, and they have always been designed to protect white people and to control Black people. Many innocent Black people are in jail because they either cannot afford bail or are forced to accept plea bargains to avoid exorbitant fines. Non-violent crimes, such as possessing small amounts of weed, can send Black men to prison for many years, stripping away their voting rights, placing them at a disadvantage in the job market, and forcing them to seek alternative ways of making a living once out of prison. Many times, those ways lead them right back to prison. It's a vicious and cruel cycle that needs to be addressed. According to the Prison Policy Initiative, the United States is responsible for 20 percent of the world's incarcerated population.

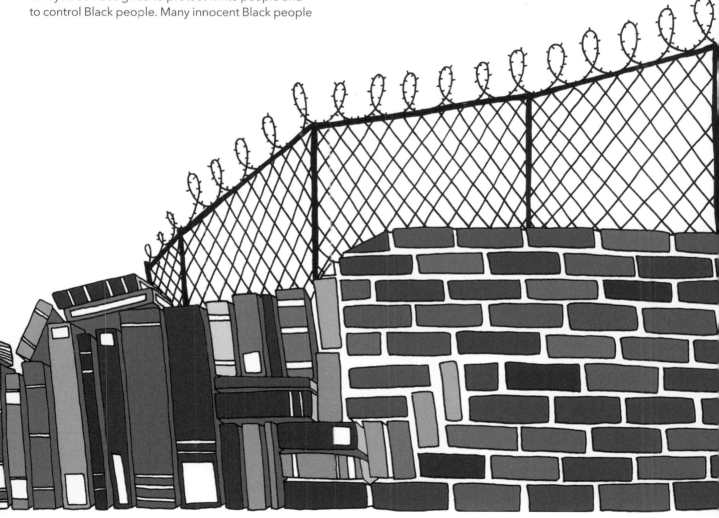

Spotlight on:

Laverne Cox

"When I was perceived as a Black man, I became a threat to public safety. When I was dressed as myself, it was my safety that was threatened."

—LAVERNE COX

Laverne Cox is a brilliant and thought-provoking speaker, Emmy-nominated actress, and documentary film producer. She has become one of the most famous transgender people in the United States. She is a recognizable (and extremely beautiful) face and an outspoken voice for LGBTQIA+ issues, particularly advocating for trans women of color.

After growing up in the dance world (primarily ballet), she began acting while at Marymount Manhattan College. It was during this time that her gender shifted from gender non-conforming to female. While in the process of transitioning, entertaining as a drag queen in New York became an outlet for both gender expression and her desire to perform. In 2007, seeing Candis Cayne become the first openly trans actor on primetime television prompted an epiphany for Cox, who realized that she could make it as a professional trans actress. In 2012, she became a household name starring in the TV show *Orange Is the New Black*.

As a prominent Black trans woman, Laverne Cox has been and will continue to be an important representative for trans people, particularly Black trans women, in mainstream media. She is a powerhouse of advocacy for trans rights and an incredible actress we all get to admire and learn from.

Cox says, "Each and every one of us has the capacity to be an oppressor. I want to encourage each and every one of us to interrogate how we might be an oppressor and how we might be able to become liberators for ourselves and for each other."

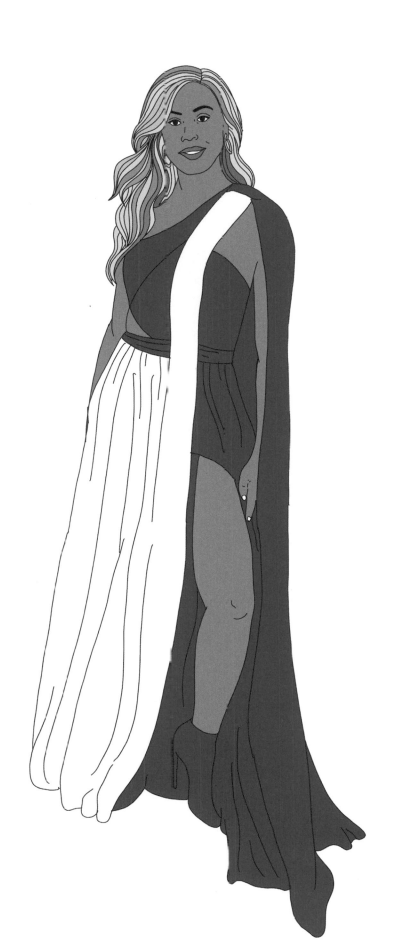

A woman sleeps with five
people in one month.

Society says: She's a slut.

A man sleeps with five
people in one month.

Society says: He's a player.

Sexual Assault, #metoo, and Gendered Violence

Sexual violence is rampant around the world, and probably has been as long as there have been humans. It has at least been around since ancient Egypt, where we can see in a script, Papyrus Salt 124, an account detailing the crimes, sexual violence, and corruption of a man named Paneb. Accounts of sexual violence are found in stories from ancient Greece, the Middle Ages, colonization in the last half century, slavery, and every war in history, by the forty-fifth US president, and in the news today.

If I were to list all of the perpetrators of sexual assault, harassment, or inappropriate/nonconsensual sexual behavior who have been publicly accused and/or legally reprimanded for their violence, the list would be thousands of pages long and continually growing.

If I were to list all of the perpetrators of sexual assault, harassment, or inappropriate/nonconsensual sexual behavior who have *not* been reported, punished, or held accountable because the criminal justice system has failed to protect the victim, the list would be hundreds and hundreds of thousands of pages long and exponentially growing.

Heartbreakingly, the topic of sexual violence could fill this whole book, and it is a source of deep sadness and anger for anyone who has either experienced this type of violence/harassment or is close to someone who has. As I see the power and pain of people stepping forward to say #metoo, I recognize how important it is to stand with and speak for others who are unable to speak for themselves. There is a deep, painful shame that often comes with being a victim of violence, and many don't speak up out of fear of risking safety, relationships, or privacy.

We are living in a moment of change, where victims of assault and harassment are stepping forward to share their experiences. It is so important that in this moment of #metoo accountability, there is transparency, truth, and bravery. And yet, we have so much further to go before the incidence of sexual violence truly shifts in a downward direction.

In 2017, after allegations against Harvey Weinstein surfaced, the #metoo movement demonstrated how rampant sexual harassment and assault are and how powerful the tool of social media can be. The phrase #metoo was coined by civil rights activist Tarana Burke as early as 2006—used in a campaign for "empowerment through empathy." *Me too* is the phrase Burke later wished she'd said to a thirteen-year-old girl who confided in her about her sexual assault. She used the phrase later to encourage solidarity and strength for women of color who have experienced abuse—a simple way to say you are not alone.

The outcomes of this movement are huge:

- Clarifying what behaviors constitute sexual harassment
- Greater awareness of the magnitude of sexual violence
- Focusing on enforcing punishment for those accused
- Promoting early education on consent and sex ed in schools
- Requiring mandatory consent classes in high school and college
- Increased effort in getting untested rape kits processed

While the hashtag has empowered some victims to make their experiences public, the flood of #metoo stories on social media feeds has been triggering to others. Constant talk of sexual violence, even for the purpose of visibility and empowerment, can be traumatizing to those who have experienced it. Keep being angry and keep fighting, but stay compassionate, conscious, and considerate of those around you who are struggling to not relive their own trauma.

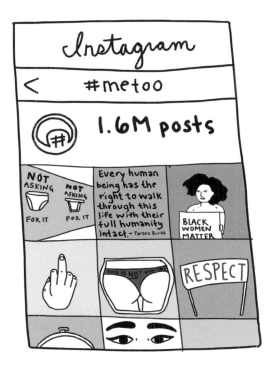

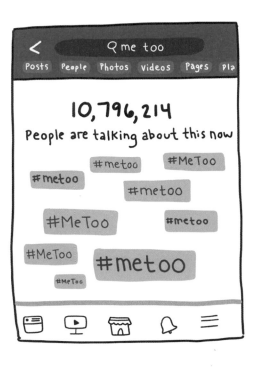

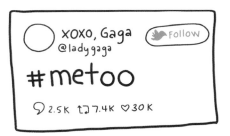

Anita Hill and Christine Blasey Ford

"Over and over I heard, 'We have a schedule, we have to press ahead with this.'. . . Are we concerned about formalities or reality? We need to value the human experience over tradition."

—ANITA HILL ON THE SENATE JUDICIARY COMMITTEE HEARING FOR SUPREME COURT NOMINEE BRETT KAVANAUGH

In October 2018, I spent several days listening to the Senate Judiciary Committee hearing for Supreme Court nominee Brett Kavanaugh, who had been accused by Dr. Christine Blasey Ford of sexual assault. One day I listened in my car for an hour in a grocery store parking lot, so upset and yet unable to turn it off or tune it out. The testimony she gave was heart-breaking. She was vulnerable, honest, strong, and nervous, and she was met with anger, hostility, and defensiveness—by both the nominated judge and the Senate.

Twenty-seven years earlier, in 1991, Anita Hill had brought sexual harassment allegations against Justice Clarence Thomas and testified to this during his nomination hearings. It was one of the first public allegations of sexual harassment brought against a man in power. It was deeply controversial and remains a foundational moment in what is now the #metoo movement. At the time, Hill was working for Thomas at the Equal Employment Opportunity Commission and alleged that the sexual misconduct happened in the workplace.

While certain elements are different between the two cases—race, political climate, how long ago the misconduct occurred, and general understanding of gendered experiences—there are eerie similarities. Kavanaugh even repeated what Thomas said word for word during his hearing: "This is a circus . . . This confirmation process has become a national disgrace." In response to the bravery of these women and disgust about their ill treatment, there has been an outpouring of support for them. In 1991, following the testimony of Anita Hill, sixteen hundred Black women pitched in money to take out a full-page ad in the *New York Times* to show public support for her. In 2018, sixteen hundred men took out an ad to show public support for both Hill and Ford.

After twenty-seven years, we now have greater awareness of trauma, sexual assault, and gender disparities, and one would think it *might* change how these women would be treated by those in power. But in a room of mostly white men, these two women were treated with suspicion and demeaned and dismissed by the majority of senators (in the Ford hearing, Republican senators). Both accused men were confirmed as judges despite the allegations; to men in power, a "he said, she said" situation will always end with "he said." It's hard to understand how far we're moving forward and how far we're sliding backward, but at the end of the day, **I believe them.**

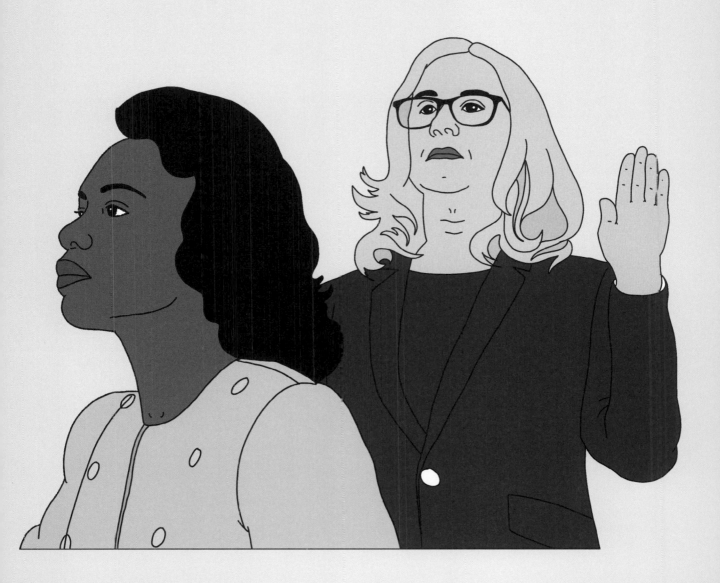

Eating Disorders Don't Discriminate

Our bodies are the focus of immense scrutiny by ourselves and others. An estimated 24 million Americans suffer from eating disorders (ED), sometimes referred to as a *silent epidemic*. We live in a culture rife with fat phobia—primarily directed at women—and a fixation on unattainable beauty standards. It's a massive issue, made worse by a lack of public discussion about the wide range of people affected by eating disorders and very limited care options for those affected.

For a start, we are shown only a sliver of the truth about how eating disorders manifest and who they affect. Anorexia and other eating disorders are usually depicted in two ways in media:

- A young, white, upper-class girl is driven by societal or parental pressures into an eating disorder. She is either trying to become more attractive (thin) to be more sexually desirable and feminine, or she's restricting out of a desire to exert control. Think *Skins*, *Pretty Little Liars*, or Betty Draper in *Mad Men*. If you search for the term *eating disorder*, almost every picture will be of a thin, young white girl.

- A middle-aged woman or unpopular girl is shown binge-eating ice cream after a breakup and is "letting herself go." This stereotype discounts overeating as a serious eating disorder and perpetuates fat phobia.

These portrayals are an inaccurate and incomplete depiction of people's struggles with eating disorders.

Men, people of color, and queer, transgender, and elderly people are just as affected by eating disorders (if not more). The mental, emotional, and physical reasons behind eating disorders can vary widely from person to person, many of which we don't think about in our usual discussions surrounding eating issues. Here are some of the reasons why someone could develop an eating disorder:

- Men who feel pressure to be more masculine/have a more muscular body can develop addictive behavior around exercise and severely restrict or alter their food intake.

- Genderqueer or transgender people who don't feel comfortable in their bodies but who aren't able or wanting to surgically change their bodies feel they can have some level of control with food or extreme exercise.

- Women who have experienced sexual assault might overeat to dissociate from trauma, make themselves feel more protected from the threat of male violence, or reduce unsolicited male attention. (Fat phobia is very directly correlated to more or less weight being deemed attractive.)

- People who have mental illnesses such as anxiety, depression, borderline personality disorder, bipolar disorder, PTSD, and OCD might be more likely to develop an eating disorder.

- Elderly people are assumed to not be as sexual or desirable as they once were, stoking self-doubt and putting huge pressure on feeling attractive and confident. One does not grow out of mental illness just because of age, and the elderly often lose consistent support networks over time.

- In certain cultures where it is rude to turn down offerings of food, one may purge in secret or restrict when alone.

- Children raised around diet culture or explicit beauty standards (such as parents with eating disorders or interest in child beauty pageants) absorb that as normal behavior for adults.

- People—particularly women of color—see only thin white women being upheld as the model for beauty standards.

- Children raised in homes where food was scarce adopt a scarcity mentality.

- Eating disorders are often genetic.

If you are not expected or "supposed" to have an illness, there is a much smaller chance you'll feel comfortable sharing your struggle and receiving help or support. Because eating disorders are the deadliest mental illness in the United States, it is vital that we begin to see people outside of the stereotypes, do not shame them, acknowledge that they are suffering, and broaden our vision of who needs and is granted access to expensive and often exclusive medical care.

And for the love of God, do not say "eat a hamburger."

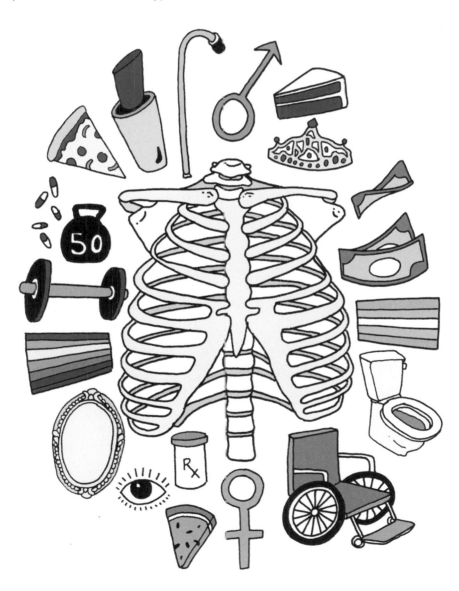

All Aging Is Not Created Equal

(or so we're told)

Men and women are not treated equally when it comes to the universal process of our bodies growing older. Luckily, we don't stop emotionally, intellectually, and socially maturing in our mid-twenties, but many people wish they could stop physically aging at their "prime." (Woof—my mid-twenties were not my prime.) We have a pretty warped idea of aging—we use creams, UV rays, face-lifts, Botox, hair plugs, and more to pretend it's not happening or hide it along the way.

While many (if not most) people have elements of self-consciousness around aging, it's women who are made to feel like their aging decreases their beauty, worth, self-confidence, and prospects for love and work. Men, on the other hand, are often seen as more dignified, wise, and powerful the older they get. We have created a world in which men are allowed to age and women are not.

Let's think for a moment about the ways in which we view boys' transition to men versus girls' transition to women. Men grow facial and body hair, get deeper voices, gain muscle mass, and develop a strong jawline. All of these things translate to power, masculinity, strength, and maturity. The feminine standard of beauty is rooted in youth: very little body hair, clear skin, perky breasts, and thinness. It is an impossible ask to expect women to remain stuck at age eighteen. A ten-year-old should look ten, a forty-year-old should look forty, and a sixty-year-old should look sixty.

There is no universal way to age; some people get wrinkles, some people lose their hair, some grow long hairs out of their ears, and others have skin that sags here and there—and **it's all okay, no matter what gender you are.**

In order to achieve aging without gender bias, we must adjust our thoughts and behavior:

- **We must make people feel valuable in their bodies no matter how they look.** A body does not inherently reflect intelligence, wisdom, strength, emotion, history, or ability. A wrinkled body is a beautiful body. A fat body is a beautiful body. A hairy body is a beautiful body—even better if some of the hair is gray. A hunched body is a beautiful body.

- **We must acknowledge that everyone ages.** The notion that one gender should age at a different speed than another gender is ridiculous. Let people age with grace, power, and dignity.

- **We must stop using advertising to encourage women to purchase youth.** This creates an unrealistic and harmful standard that women feel pressured to achieve. Women already get paid less per hour on the whole; don't try to trick women into spending their lower-than-men's hourly wage on products based largely on the beauty standards set by men.

We must try hard to undo our internalized ageism, particularly when it comes to beauty standards and older women. We unknowingly judge people based on their perceived age all the time, whether in hiring practices, internet dating, or friendship. The older someone gets, the more capable and wiser they'll likely be—even about things you'd expect them not to be. Be humble, youth; your elders have learned something along the way.

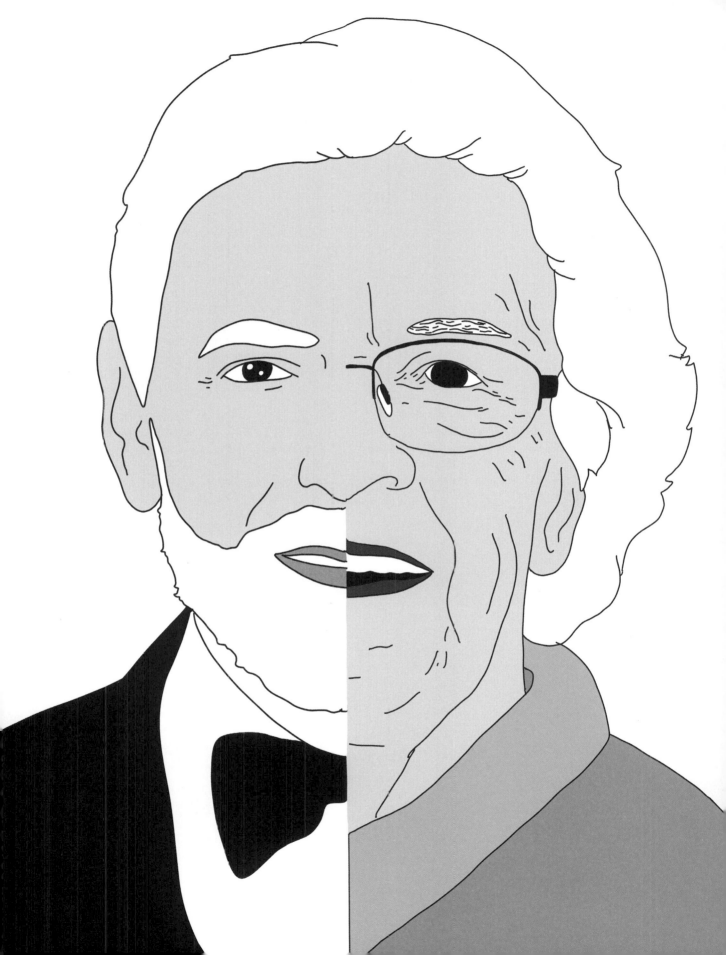

Abortion

Abortion is an essential human rights issue and fundamentally grants people assigned female at birth (AFAB) the choice of bodily freedom, reproductive decisions, family planning, and privacy.

Note: I'm going to use the acronym AFAB to describe anyone who needs access to abortion care. However, I want to acknowledge that intersex people that have varying sex assignments at birth are also able to get pregnant. Many genders can get pregnant and need to have comprehensive reproductive rights—cis women, genderqueer people, trans men, and intersex people.

"When women are compelled to carry and bear children, they are subjected to 'involuntary servitude' in violation of the Thirteenth Amendment. . . . [Even] if the woman has stipulated to have consented to the risk of pregnancy, that does not permit the state to force her to remain pregnant."

–ANDREW KOPPELMAN, "FORCED LABOR: A THIRTEENTH AMENDMENT DEFENSE OF ABORTION"

Roe v. Wade was a seminal moment in the second-wave feminism fight for women's rights, granting in 1973 the right to legally have an abortion. Justified by the court as "right to privacy," abortion was granted as a decision to be made by the person who is pregnant. However, there were limitations set in place. During the first trimester, it is completely up to the pregnant person to terminate the pregnancy. In the second trimester, an abortion is legal only with consent from the state to determine if the procedure would negatively impact the health of the mother/birth giver. Third-trimester abortions—those after the point of fetal viability—are highly regulated and often not allowed, unless birth would endanger the mother/birth giver. Many scholars and lawyers debate about the constitutionality of legal abortion, arguing that it was not focused narrowly enough under the issue of privacy, that it is based more on the decision-making power of the doctor than the woman, and that the language surrounding viability is vague and subjective.

Opposition to abortion is usually based on the "right to life" of a fetus, or the notion that life or personhood begins at the moment of conception. Ironically, the plaintiff in *Roe v. Wade*, Norma McCorvey, became a pro-life proponent after the trial, fervently opposing abortion, citing the emotional suffering caused by abortions (hers in particular).

The history of abortion has been divisive, to say the least. It is one of the most common platforms on which political candidates run, often being a dividing factor in their voter base. The amount of control that governments have varies with the political powers over time. In some states, there are only a few clinics that provide abortions, and in some states, only one. This makes access incredibly difficult for people who live far away, do not have time off work, have children to take care of, or don't have enough money to make the trip. Spousal consent to the abortion has often been legally required, and punishment for illegal abortions has ranged from charges of manslaughter (for the death of the aborted fetus) to government shutdowns of abortion clinics to banning state funding for clinics to forcing women to watch fetal ultrasounds before allowing their abortions.

I recognize and respect that people have the right to make medical decisions regarding their own bodies. **Abortion is a legitimate and medically necessary choice for a number of reasons:**

- Unintentional pregnancy
- An inability to financially or physically care for a child
- Cultural or religious values
- Not being emotionally ready to have a child
- Pregnancy due to sexual assault
- Health complications
- An unstable relationship
- Family pressure
- Fear and shame

Remember, many states enforce abstinence-only sex education, and birth control is not thoroughly taught in some schools. Making abortion illegal or restrictive puts some people at risk for unsafe abortions and for traumatic or difficult pregnancies or births. Forcing a person to have a baby they can't afford can put them into a critical financial position or even poverty, a cycle that will continue for their children.

Most health legislation is determined by white, straight, cis men who most certainly have never experienced the process of creating a baby in your body, let alone the pain of giving birth.

In the very simplest of terms, let people decide if they want a child or are able to have one.

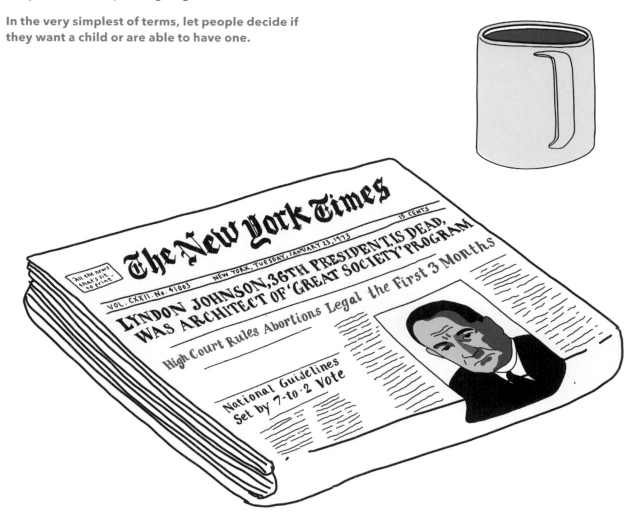

Medical Bias

Medical study results—and therefore medical treatments—are biased toward men.

Most medical institutions do not have gender participation requirements for a number of reasons, and more men participate in clinical trials than women, skewing data in potentially dangerous ways.

Drugs are prescribed at a dosage that is safe for men (based on average physical makeup and drug response) but often too high for women. Technology for heart disease is based on male-driven data, though heart problems manifest very differently in women who have just as much heart disease (it's the #1 killer of women). Study results are lumped into one group, eliminating potentially vital information that will affect sexes differently.

Currently and historically, medical studies and treatments have focused on white participants and patients. POC are often left out of studies completely or are subjects of medical malpractice and mistreatment, lowering their access to and quality of care. Most recently, POC faced a higher death rate due to COVID-19 for a wide variety of reasons ranging from access to medical facilities, higher rates of chronic medical conditions, language barriers, access to transportation, and a higher impact because of essential jobs that oftentimes do not pay for sick leave. In order to give equal medical care, we must collect medical data equally.

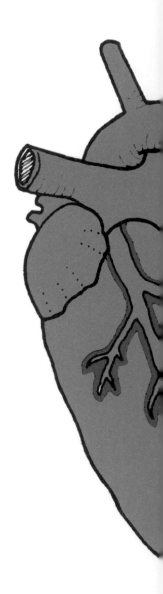

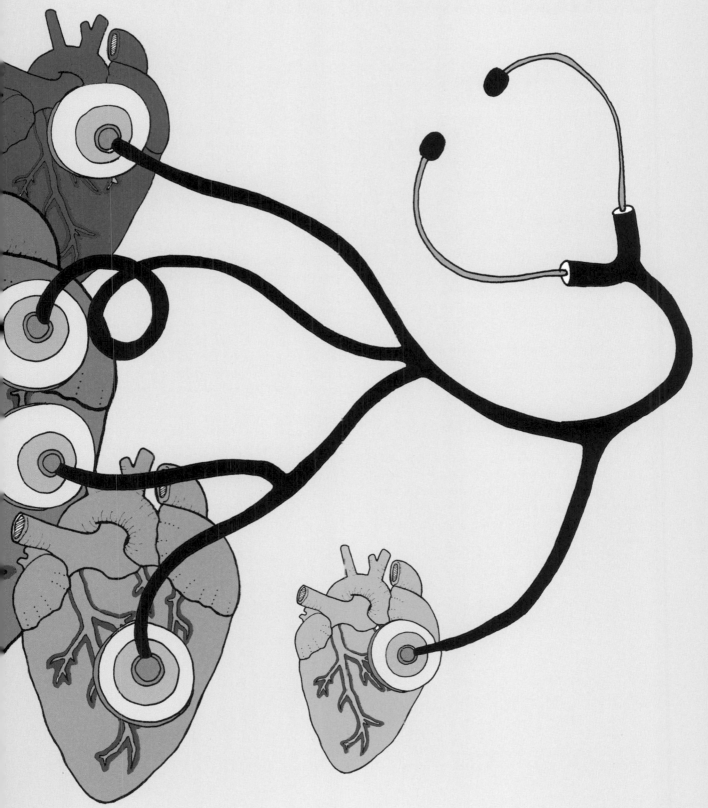

Gender and Mental Illness

Let's take depression as an example. Picture someone who is depressed. I'll bet most of you imagined a woman, not a man. According to statistics, women are twice as likely as men to develop depression (either chronic or episodic) at some point in their lives. This may be true; however, the scale on which these statistics are measured might be flawed.

In 2013, Lisa Martin and other researchers created a "gender-inclusive depression scale," which used more prevalent male symptoms like anger, substance use, risk-taking, and irritability to reduce the gender bias in studies about depression. By using a scale that included a wider range of depression symptoms experienced by all genders, they found that 30.6 percent of men and 33.3 percent of women met the criteria for depression.

There are different schools of thought about this gender disparity (or lack thereof). On one hand, women experience systemic hardship on a much grander scale: greater likelihood of trauma, fewer economic resources, stressful work and home responsibilities, postpartum depression, and often single parenthood. There is no way to separate these life conditions from mental health—they are undeniably linked and often lead to other mental and physical illnesses. Due to social circumstances and systemic gender disparities, women are more likely to experience this type of emotional and physical overworking.

On the other hand, social gender norms may discourage men from reporting their experiences with depression, skewing the data in a way that underrepresents depression in men. There is not much space created for men to cry, ask for help, or show sadness. As with many facets of masculinity, their experiences are filtered through the hegemonic norms of "manliness." More vulnerable emotions are often expressed through anger, aggression, substance abuse, gambling/risk-taking, or violence. We then categorize these as anger issues, alcoholism, promiscuity, or being a player rather than seeing them as manifestations of depression or anxiety. While abusive behaviors might be expressions of sadness, emptiness, or discontent, there isn't an excuse for that behavior—ever. But if we as a society can reduce the stigma of male vulnerability, more men may seek treatment for mental health issues. White men account for seven of ten suicides in the United States and men on the whole are three and a half times more likely to die by suicide than women.

Feeling isolated in an experience can be even more dangerous than the experience itself. We need to make it known that mental illness affects everyone and talk about how it affects populations both differently and similarly.

* The majority of studies have been focused on cis women and cis men. See "Mental Health in the Trans Community" on page 134.

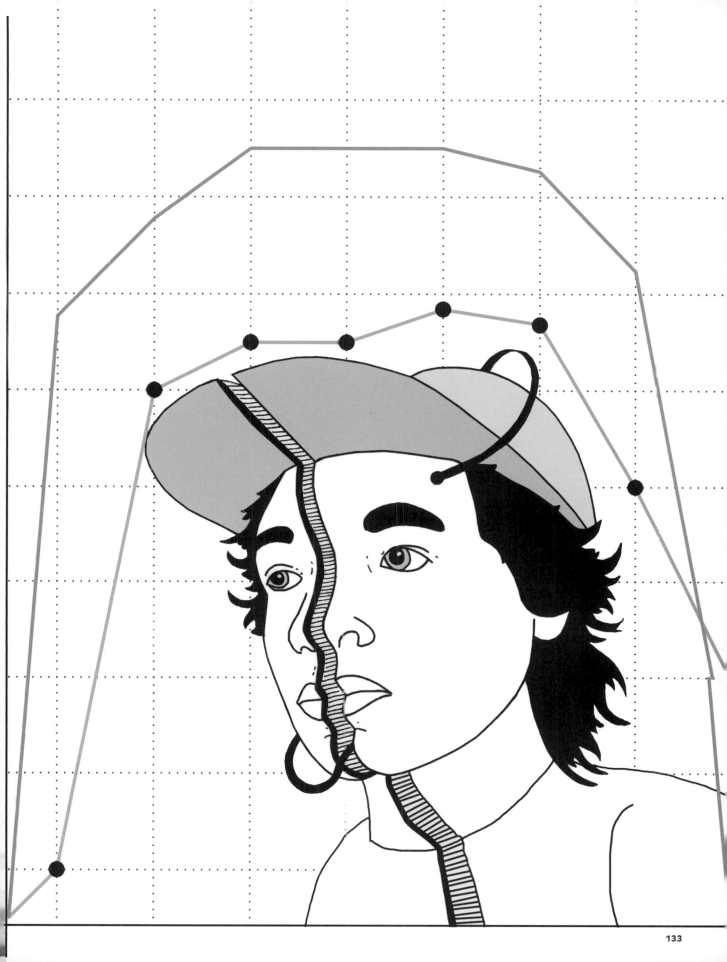

Mental Health in the Trans Community

Despite all of the amazing parts of embodying a gender that's different than your assigned sex—community, fun, fashion, acceptance, love, humor—being transgender can be really hard, dangerous, lonely, and scary.

Transgender people are at a much higher risk of psychological distress, mental health issues, bullying, sexual violence, murder, and suicide than cisgender people. In most of the United States and much of the world, being transgender is still not safe, despite growing acceptance and visibility. Religion, geographical tradition, conservative legislation, class values, homophobia, and fear can create hostility and hate.

The following disturbing stats about life (and death) as a transgender person come from the Williams Institute at UCLA, as of 2014–2015:

- 40% of trans people have attempted suicide
- 77% of trans people experienced some form of mistreatment in school, including verbal harassment (54%) and physical harassment (17%)
- 15% of respondents who had a job in the past year were verbally harassed, physically attacked, and/or sexually assaulted at work (1%)
- 23% of those who had a job in the past year reported other forms of mistreatment

- 26% reported that an immediate family member stopped speaking to them/ended their relationship altogether because they were transgender
- 10% experienced violence from a family member, and 8% were kicked out of their family home
- 33% had a negative experience with a health-care provider in the past year related to being transgender, and 3% had medical professionals refuse to treat them
- 13% experienced sexual violence in grades K–12 because of being transgender
- 30% of trans people have experienced homelessness, 12% in the last year
- 58% experienced some form of police mistreatment including verbal harassment, repeated misgendering, physical assault, or sexual assault (no specific breakdown)

Statistics about violence against the trans community are sobering and illuminate how far we have to go in making the world feel safe for people of all genders. For resources, see page 196.

YOU ARE NOT ALONE

Privilege 101

How You Might Have a Gender Advantage and Not Know It

Most people know if they have more or fewer advantages than other groups of people, whether or not they use the words *privilege* and *oppression* to describe those dynamics. Oftentimes it's much easier for us to see the oppression of others than our own privileges. If you don't see something as a problem, you probably aren't experiencing it because you have certain privilege. Being told that you are privileged can elicit negative reactions in people such as:

- "But I'm poor."
- "But my life is too hard to be privileged."
- "But I worked hard to get to where I am."
- "But I don't have it easier than _____."
- "But I'm [part of a marginalized group]."

Oppression and privilege are not mutually exclusive. All of those things can be true, and you can still have an inherent societal advantage over others. In essence, any group of people that benefits from having a certain identity has privilege. We all hold many identities, and most of us have certain aspects of advantage and disadvantage within our experience. Race, class, gender, religion, language, age, ability, and sexual orientation are some identity markers that can grant or deny privilege.

When it comes to gender, there are certain identities that move through the world with more ease than others. Some questions to ask yourself when considering your own gender privilege are:

- Do I have to worry about safety when I use a school or public restroom? Do I have to worry which restroom is safest?
- Can I show my nipples on the beach?
- Do I rely on my partner to do most of the household chores?
- Do I see myself represented in media? What are the characteristics of the people in media who look like me?
- Is my pay equal to my (equally qualified) colleague of the opposite/a different gender? Would I raise the issue to my boss if I make less? How about if I make more?
- Are the boys in my classes treated differently or given more attention, particularly in STEM subjects?
- Do I feel safe walking alone at night?
- Am I comfortable being assertive? At work? With my partner? In a classroom? With my teachers?
- Am I told to smile more?

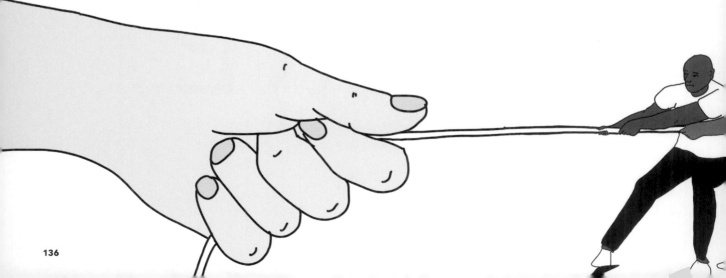

- Do I have to use my sick days or miss school for menstrual cramps?

- Can I wear whatever I want and not be catcalled? Will my outfit be used as an excuse for people to harass or assault me?

- What would people think if they were to find out I am a single parent?

- Do I feel aware of when I am loud? When I take up significant physical space? When I interrupt?

- Will the world treat me as more invisible or more powerful as I age? Do I feel the need to use products to meet a standard of attractiveness as I age?

If you don't encounter these things as problems or obstacles in your life, you most likely have some amount of privilege. Think about those who experience the fear, discomfort, or imposed limitations of their genders in these scenarios and try to come up with ways to use your privilege to alleviate the oppression of others. Here are some ways you can:

- If you own a business, give all of your qualified employees equal wages and maternity and paternity leave. Make your restrooms gender neutral, which could be as simple as labeling your bathrooms either "stalls" or "stalls and urinals," which gives each patron the choice of personal comfort regardless of gender. If you can't do that for whatever reason, designate a private locking bathroom as gender neutral.

- If you're in a meeting or a classroom discussion, be aware of how much space you're taking up with your voice and opinions. Let others in the room say their ideas and don't interrupt. Men are generally listened to more even if their ideas are no better than their female/other gender counterparts.

- If you are a white woman, do research about intersectional feminism and the experience of POC women. If you are cisgender, consider donating to trans-led organizations.

- If you are a relatively healthy man, consider donating your paid sick days to someone who needs them. Women and single mothers often use sick time, vacation days, or unpaid hours to deal with non-optional personal or family issues (sick kid, school meeting, period cramps).

- Do. Not. Catcall. Women.

- Help around the house without being asked.

We can't get rid of our unearned privilege, but we can act in a way that's less harmful to those who don't have the same privileges and use our privilege to demand equitable treatment for those around us.

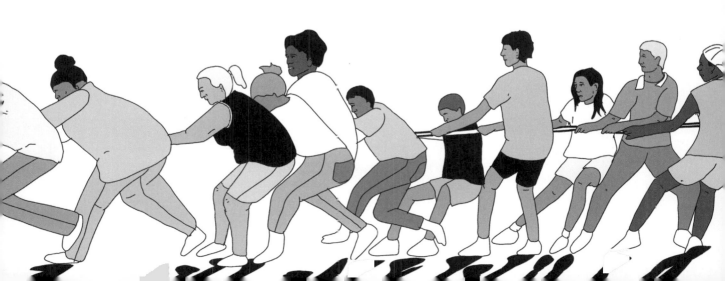

Equality ≠ Equity

The same inputs do not necessarily produce fair outcomes.

Even if you give a marginalized individual or population the same rights, resources, or opportunities as non-marginalized groups, it won't erase preexisting systems of discrimination and historical disadvantage.

The concept of equity considers the unique resources an individual or population needs in order to succeed. This acknowledges people have different needs; oppressed groups need more resources to have the same opportunities as those who aren't oppressed.

One common example of the disparity between equality and equity is in the classroom. Students with learning differences and disabilities are often given the exact same resources as kids without similar difficulties—same teacher, same lessons, same levels of attention, and same pace of learning. This often does not create equitable outcomes, and instead gives students without learning disabilities a systemic advantage in traditional school systems. Without specialized attention, the ability to have different methods of learning, or slower-paced lessons, those with learning disabilities will struggle both in and after school.

True equality means meeting varied needs in varied ways.

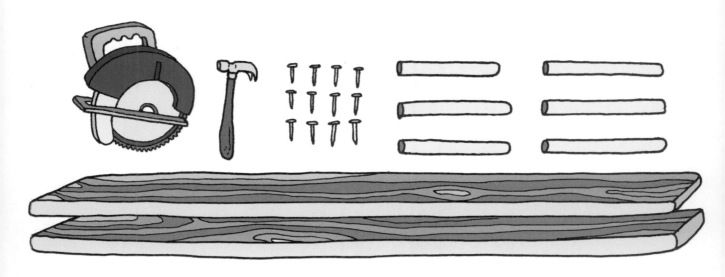

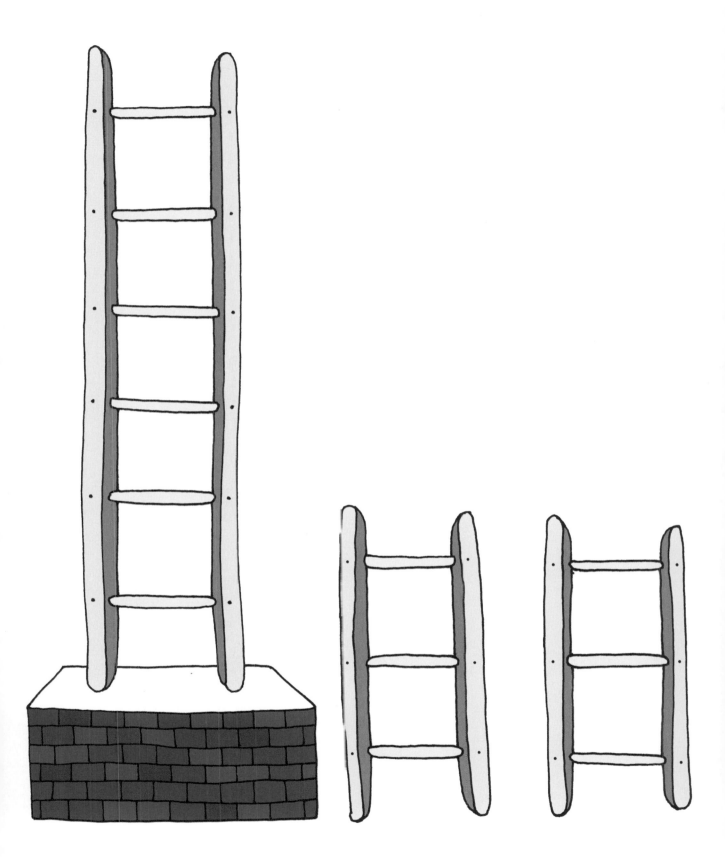

Pink Tax

Women, on average, pay 7 percent more than men for the same products with different marketing.

- For personal care products, women pay 13% more than men.
- For clothing, women pay 8% more than men.
- Girls' toys cost 7% more than boys' toys.
- Girls' clothing costs 4% more than boys'.

And don't forget service discrepancies; from haircuts to dry cleaning and even mortgage interest, women pay more for many things than men do.

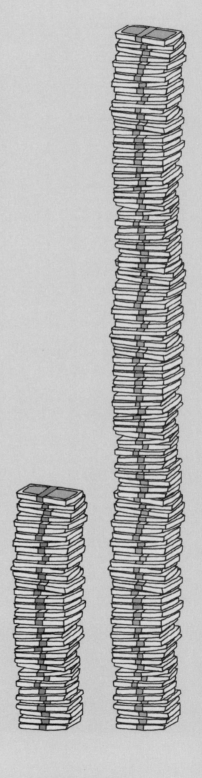

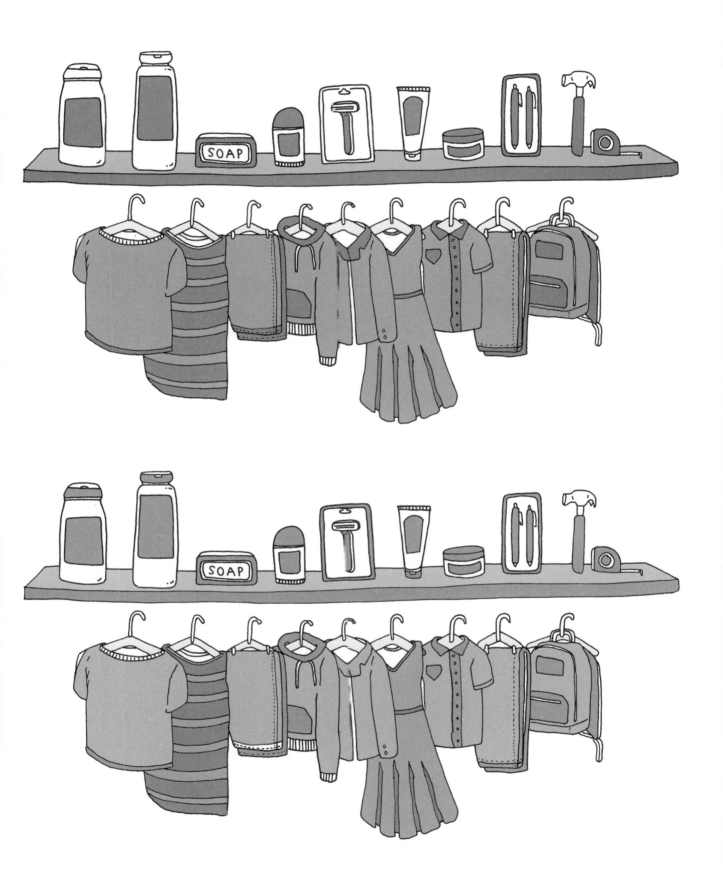

Feminization of Poverty

Women represent a disproportionate percentage of the world's poor. Poverty's effects can extend beyond lack of financial wealth into poverty of opportunity, health, education, safety, decision-making power in households or government, basic freedom and human rights, and resources.

Single mothers around the globe are the most at-risk population for extreme poverty due to many factors: lower-paying jobs (because of the global gender-wage gap), a single income, no health-care or employee benefits for part-time work, housing instability, or lack of access to healthy and consistent meals. On top of this large-scale inequity, single mothers are responsible for basic household labor and emotional support as the primary caregiver to their families. When some or all of these factors combine, it creates an uphill battle to achieve financial, emotional, and domestic stability for single mothers and their children.

Global statistics are hard to confirm because most statistics are an amalgamation of several organizations' research with different methods and scopes.* However, the worldwide pattern of poverty is clear:

- The international poverty line is $1.90 a day.

- In 2016 there were 40.6 million people in poverty in the United States (12.3% of the population).

- Globally, on average, women earn 23% less than men and are 38% more likely to live in poverty than men.

- 75% of women in developing regions work in the informal economy (jobs or work not taxed or regulated by the state).

- 14% of children in the world live in single-family households, 80% headed by women. Over half of these children live under the poverty line.

- In 2014, 30.6% of single female-headed families lived in poverty, three times higher than families with two parents.

- Childcare costs are 103.6% of a single parent's minimum wage income in Washington, DC ($22,631 for one year of infant care; $21,840 full-time minimum wage salary).

- 10:1 is the wealth ratio of white families to Black families.

- 122 women between the ages of 25 and 34 live in poor households for every 100 men of the same age group.

*Data from Organisation for Economic Cooperation and Development (36 countries), US Census, World Bank (89 countries), and Oxfam.

The 2016 US population:

- 76.6% white
- 13.4% Black
- 18.1% Latinx
- 5.8% Asian
- 1.3% Native American

The percentage of women in poverty:

- 9.7% white
- 21.4% Black
- 18.7% Latinx
- 10.7% Asian
- 22.8% Native American

The percentage of children in poverty:

- 10.8% white
- 30.8% Black
- 26.6% Latinx
- 11.1% Asian
- 25.4% Native American

The percentage of households headed by a single mother:

- 15% white
- 49% Black
- 26% Latinx
- 11% Asian
- 10.2% Native American

The percentage of households headed by a single mother in poverty:

- 30.2% white
- 38.3% Black
- 40.8% Latinx
- 20.0% Asian
- 42.6% Native American

Spotlight on:

The Zapatistas

The Zapatista Army of National Liberation (EZLN) is a leftist indigenous group in Chiapas, one of the poorest states in Mexico. The group began as a secret organization with a mission to protect rural communities in Mexico through peaceful tactics but violence when necessary. The women in Chiapas, the Zapatistas, have historically had very few rights, all of which were contained within their home rather than in public or governing bodies. However, in the last three decades they have created a self-sustaining infrastructure that prioritizes women's rights and gives much of the decision-making power to women.

The Zapatistas passed the Women's Revolutionary Law, which was published in January 1994. It states:

1. Women, regardless of their race, creed, color, or political affiliation, have the right to participate in the revolutionary struggle in any way that their desire and capacity determine.

2. Women have the right to work and receive a fair salary.

3. Women have the right to decide the number of children they have and care for.

4. Women have the right to participate in the matters of the community and hold office if they are free and democratically elected.

5. Women and their children have the right to primary attention in their health and nutrition.

6. Women have the right to an education.

7. Women have the right to choose their partner and are not obliged to enter into marriage.

8. Women have the right to be free of violence from both relatives and strangers.

9. Women will be able to occupy positions of leadership in the organization and hold military ranks in the revolutionary armed forces.

10. Women will have all the rights and obligations elaborated in the Revolutionary Laws and regulations.

One of the factors that made these laws even more possible to maintain was the banning of alcohol (and drugs), a ban that still remains in place today. Eliminating alcohol from their society greatly reduced domestic violence against women and kept the little money available with the people of the EZLN.

The essential underpinning of the EZLN was that women's rights within their community were integrated with their fight for rights and recognition from the Mexican government—they recognized that women's rights were necessary for the larger fight to succeed. When Comandanta Ramona (one of the leaders and founders of the EZLN) passed away, it was said by fellow member Subcomandante Marcos that "the world has lost one of those women who gives birth to new worlds."

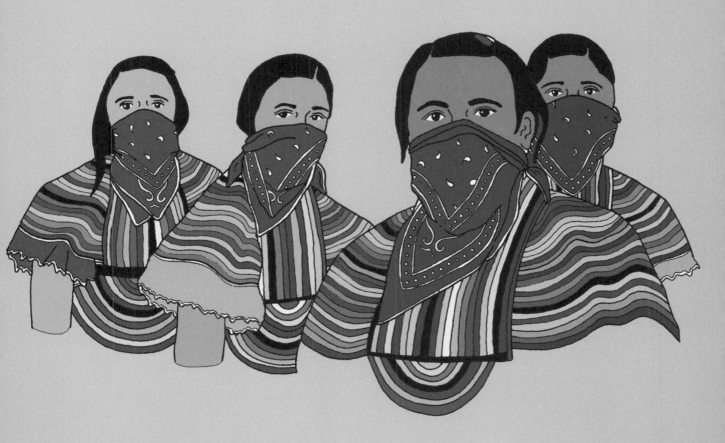

The Quiet Southern Epidemic

HIV/AIDS in Black and Latino Gay Male Communities

The AIDS epidemic of the 1980s was one of the most prominent medical, political, and social issues of the time. It ravaged gay communities, killing huge numbers of homosexual and bisexual men, as well as intravenous drug users and sex workers. However, access to information and health care was, and still is, disproportionately divided between people of different races, classes, and geographic regions.

After the fight against AIDS in the '80s led to the development of HIV drugs that inhibit the disease's progression to AIDS, many thought that the HIV/AIDS crisis was mostly under control. **This assumption is not only incorrect, but dangerous.** The southern United States is now home to the highest percentage of people diagnosed with HIV in the United States, accounting for 50 percent of new HIV infections in 2016.

HIV transmission rates between Black and Latino men who have sex with men (MSM) are high: one in two Black men and one in four Latino men will contract HIV through sexual encounters with men in their lifetime. Many MSMs do not self-identify as gay or queer. While the Center for Disease Control and Prevention (CDC) studies did not specify these figures were for the South, it does acknowledge the South has the highest rate of HIV transmission in the United States.

These high rates are both caused and influenced by factors such as inadequate sex education, conservative legislation, and religious and institutional homophobia. Along with limited financial and medical resources for treatment, these factors present significant barriers to obtaining both preventative care (to curb the rate of infection) and treatment if infected.

Undocumented Latino men face additional issues: They may not be able to seek treatment due to citizenship status or lack of insurance, and even if they do, they may not speak English well, if at all. Disclosing sexual history is already an incredibly intimate act, and a language barrier could further inhibit the sharing of deeply personal information.

In this region, where queer and gay identities are still widely stigmatized, there exists a culture of shame and secrecy. I grew up and currently live in the South, where schools more often than not teach abstinence-only sex ed. In an environment that doesn't even acknowledge straight sex, imagine how difficult it must be for someone to safely have queer sex and get access to medical and mental health treatment related to their sexual orientation.

The South is the most religious part of the United States. While in many religious communities being out as LGBTQIA+ or HIV positive is very difficult, an individual's spirituality/religion has been shown to have positive effects on health outcomes/treatment among Black and Latino MSM.

HIV statistics in the United States as of 2016 according to the CDC:

- Since 1981, 1,232,246 people have been diagnosed with AIDS.

- 63% of HIV infections occur in MSM populations.

- 18.5 per 100,000 people have HIV in the South (higher than any other region in the United States).

- Black MSM and gay men have the highest rate of HIV in the United States, accounting for 55% of new infections among young MSM.

- 21% of new HIV diagnoses are Latinos, with MSM accounting for 85% of those.

These statistics are sobering to say the least, and hopefully the more this issue is brought to light, the more potential it has to change for the better.

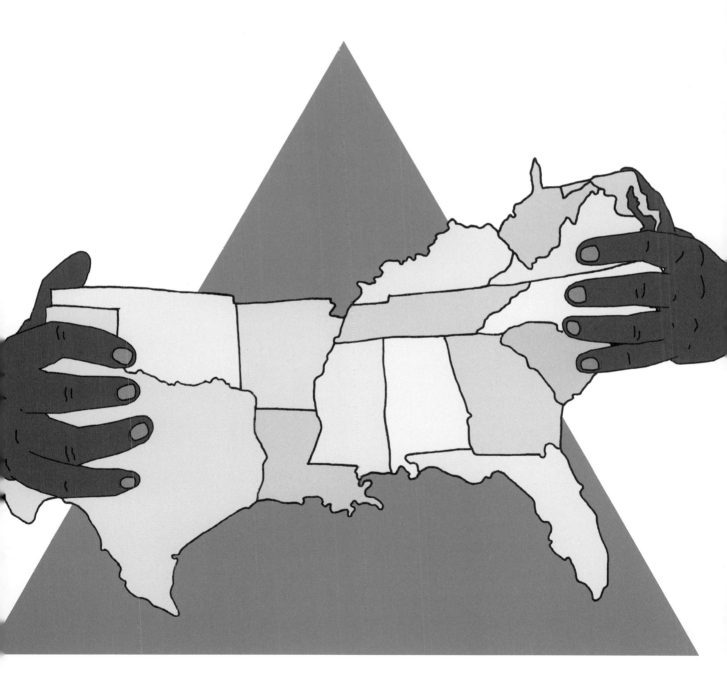

The Public Facilities Privacy & Security Act

(HB2 Bill)

There are countless ways that governments have discriminated against queer, trans, and gender-non-conforming people, including the Public Facilities Privacy & Security Act passed in 2016 in North Carolina, which prohibits people from using public bathrooms that align with their gender, and forces them to use the bathroom for the gender listed on their birth certificate. This means transgender men would be forced to use women's bathrooms and vice versa.

"Local boards of education shall require every multiple occupancy bathroom or changing facility that is designated for student use to be designated for and used only by students based on their biological sex."

–PUBLIC FACILITIES PRIVACY & SECURITY ACT, GENERAL ASSEMBLY OF NORTH CAROLINA

Let me pause on this absurd law, as it deserves some analysis and is very personal to me as a genderqueer North Carolina native who is routinely stared at in the bathroom. The law claims to be protective, but it is simply, and deeply, transphobic. Setting aside the meat of their argument, prohibiting anyone from using a public facility to meet a basic need is discriminatory and wrong. Governments should not be controlling bathroom usage in an effort to exert gender bias.

The lawmakers behind HB2 claim the primary reason for the law is the fear that transgender women (who in their eyes are men) are using the women's bathroom only for predatory purposes that put cisgender women in danger. However, being a visible trans woman using a men's bathroom can be incredibly scary, and oftentimes, quite dangerous. The bill that claims to be an effort to protect women is putting trans women in danger. Enforcing this law forces trans men to use women's bathrooms. So, instead of allowing people to use the bathroom with people who look like them, the law is doing the opposite and inviting men (yes, trans men are men) to use the women's bathroom—the exact issue they were fearing.

Using a public bathroom is a basic human right. Let people choose the bathroom of their comfort without question.

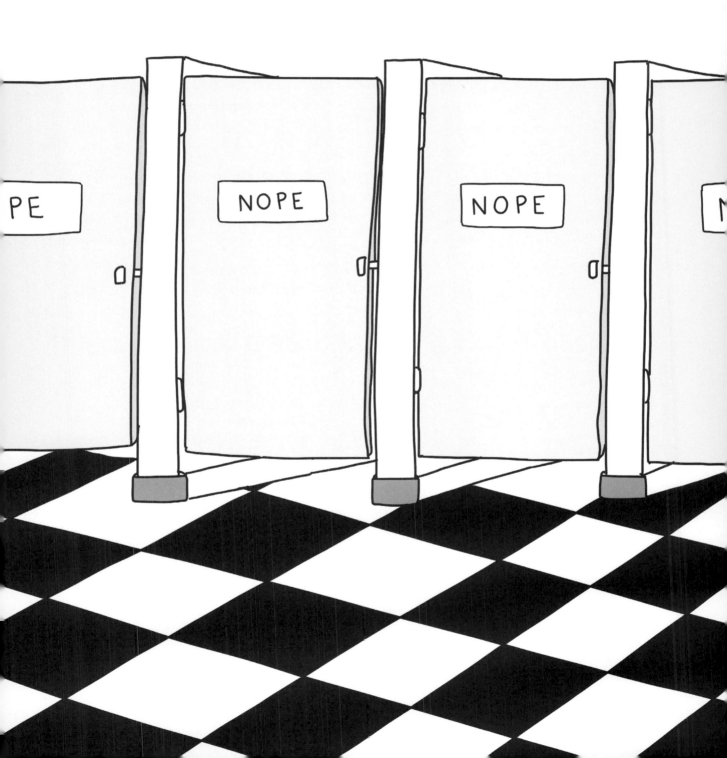

Sex Work Is Not a Bad Term

"'Sex work' is a broad term used to describe exchanges of sex or sexual activity. Sex work is also used as a non-stigmatizing term for 'prostitution.' . . . Using the term 'sex work' reinforces the idea that sex work is work and allows for greater discussion of labor rights and conditions. Not every person in the sex trade defines themselves as a sex worker or their sexual exchange as work. Some may not regard what they do as labor at all, but simply a means to get what they need. Others may be operating within legal working conditions, such as pornography or exotic dancing, and wish to avoid the negative associations with illegal or informal forms of sex work. In addition to the exchange of money for sexual services, a person may exchange sex or sexual activity for things they need or want, such as food, housing, hormones, drugs, gifts, or other resources. 'Survival sex' is a term used by many nonprofit organizations and researchers to describe trading of sex for survival needs."

–"MEANINGFUL WORK: TRANSGENDER EXPERIENCES IN THE SEX TRADE," 2015, BY ERIN FITZGERALD, SARAH ELSPETH PATTERSON, AND DARBY HICKEY (WITH CHERNO BIKO AND HARPER JEAN TOBIN)

Sex work is one of the oldest jobs in history, if not *the* oldest. Transactional sex in one form or another has been practiced since ancient times. Over time, sex work has shifted from something common and even celebrated to something highly stigmatized.

One important thing to note is that sex work is work. It's a job like being a store clerk, an architect, or a freelance writer. We all, unfortunately, have to do work to make a living. Some of us hate our jobs and some of us love them—the same goes for those who do sex work. Sadly, sex work is generally misunderstood, judged, and criminalized, and it's often dangerous for those who do it regardless of whether it's out of enjoyment, necessity, or both. It's important not to conflate sex work and sex trafficking; there's a vital difference between the two. Sex work is a consensual exchange between adults; sex trafficking

is a human rights violation that uses violence, abduction, or coercion to sexually exploit vulnerable people. Sex workers do not condone sex trafficking.

Sex work is a very divisive issue—some believe it perpetuates oppression, sexual violence, and the commodification of women's bodies, while others believe sex work is a legitimate form of work and that consensual sexual expression should not be vilified for going against heteronormative standards. It's a complicated subject and is closely tied to intersectionality. The reasons one might have for getting into this line of work and the experiences they might have can vary widely depending on race, gender, class, geographical region, and mental health. Positions range from high-end escorts who can pull in half a million dollars a year to street workers who can barely make ends meet.

Sex workers who are people of color are more at risk of being the victims of sexual and emotional violence. This is particularly true for trans women of color, drug users, and undocumented individuals who go into sex work when housing and jobs are inaccessible due to gender discrimination and systemic disadvantage. It can be dangerous work. According to a 2012 study by Kathleen N. Deering et al., sex workers have a 45 to 75 percent chance of experiencing sexual violence in their careers at the hands of clients, pimps, and law enforcement. Because almost all sex work is criminalized, there is very little access to necessary health and social services, and very few legal protections for the rights of those who do the work. In addition, it's difficult for victims of violence and rape to report it without being arrested themselves.

There are several models used all over the world for legalizing/decriminalizing sex work with various levels of success, from Nevada in the United States (legalized brothels with safety procedures built in) to decriminalizing sex work but making it illegal to buy sexual services (Canada). In theory, the latter model gives the seller full agency to determine their working conditions, but they must be covert about their work and therefore it reinforces underground sex work.

Whether you agree with it or not, sex work exists everywhere. And because it exists, those who do it must be granted basic human rights to access medical care, legal action for cases of sexual violence, safe housing, and acknowledgment that what they do is actually work. It's important to suspend judgment and bias for those in this line of work and begin to talk about it in a non-stigmatized way.

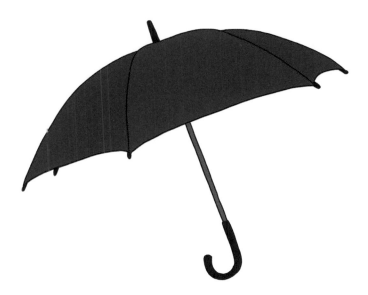

⌃THE RED UMBRELLA IS THE WORLDWIDE SYMBOL OF THE SEX WORKERS' RIGHTS MOVEMENT

Spotlight on:
The Stonewall Uprising
(June 28, 1969)

1961: Homosexuality is criminalized—not explicitly illegal—in all states except Illinois. Illinois is the first state to "decriminalize homosexual acts" by repealing sodomy laws in 1961.

June 28, 1969, 1:20 A.M.: A revolutionary moment in queer history.

At the time in New York City, gay bars had gotten approval (since 1966) to obtain liquor licenses, but police raids were still common because people could still be arrested for "gay behaviors" such as kissing, touching, contact dancing, and cross-dressing. The Stonewall Inn was one of the few bars where people could dance openly. The Stonewall Inn wasn't just a bar, it was a safe social and community space for queer, homeless transgender youth, and drag queens to go at a time when most gay bars wouldn't allow people in drag to enter, and there weren't community centers for youths rendered homeless by familial rejection.

On the heels of many other gay bars being shut down, the routine police raid of June 28 turned into a six-day riot, when Stonewall patrons refused to go quietly. After a woman being violently arrested yelled, "Why don't you guys do something?" the growing crowd of bystanders did something. Police had always operated on the wrong assumption that the queer community wouldn't fight back—that shame and fear would prevent them from outing themselves through protest, or that gay men were too effeminate, weak, and passive to ever fight back. By the second night, more than a thousand people had gathered in protest.

Michael Fader, a patron involved in the riots said, "There was something in the air, freedom a long time overdue, and we're going to fight for it. It took different forms, but the bottom line was, we weren't going to go away. And we didn't."

For six days, the area near Stonewall saw thrown rocks, chanting drag queens, police hitting protesters, protesters hitting police, protesters rocking cars trying to drive by, a parking meter used as a battering ram, garbage can fires, and can-can dances. Queer people can make a good dance party anywhere.

The Stonewall riots finally ended, but the event sparked the start of the public gay rights movement and birthed the Gay Liberation Front, the Gay Activists Alliance, and the first Gay Pride parade, held the year after the riots (known in that year as the Christopher Street Liberation Day).

June 26, 2003: Homosexuality is decriminalized in the final fourteen states (Virginia, North Carolina, South Carolina, Alabama, Florida, Mississippi, Missouri, Utah, Louisiana, Texas, Oklahoma, Idaho, Kansas, and Michigan).

June 24, 2016: The Stonewall Inn is designated as a US National Monument, the first to be dedicated to LGBTQIA+ history.

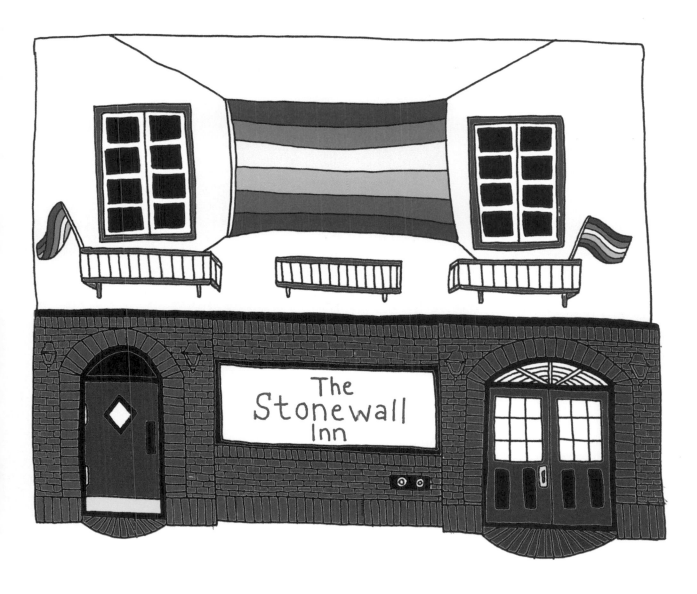

LGBTQ+ Is Not a Monolith

"Honestly, I hate to admit it, but I'm not immersed in the gay community. Therefore, I'm ignorant. I don't know the correct pronouns . . . I feel fucking stupid, quite honestly. I've always looked at trans people and I've thought, 'Why don't you just—? Like it costs so much, and it can be really painful. Why put yourself through that?' It seems quite a traumatic experience. I truly didn't understand what that meant to actually have the surgery done and feel that change. There are so many people out there like me, who are ignorant, who don't understand. I think that probably most straight people assume that because it's LGBTQ+, we must all understand each other's plight. But that couldn't be more wrong."

–TAN FRANCE OF *QUEER EYE*, IN CONVERSATION WITH SKYLER, A TRANSGENDER MAN FEATURED IN SEASON 2, EPISODE 5

There is a common misconception among both straight and queer people that all sectors of the LGBTQIA+ community overlap, interact, or share space regularly. This isn't true in most circumstances. I cannot speak for everyone, but in my life as a queer person I am not around gay men, two-spirit people, or people who identify as lesbian; I am around lots of people who identify as cis women, genderqueer, and trans* (see note).

Note: *Some use trans* (with an asterisk) as an umbrella term for all non-cisgender identities. However, trans (without an asterisk) usually refers to people who identify as transgender.*

It makes sense. Most groups of people who fit into an umbrella category of any sort generally do not interact with every other sector of that same identity, and that's really okay. So be aware that when you speak with someone in the LGBTQIA+ community, they may not be personally familiar with the experiences of others in that same wide community. There is room to grow and understand a huge variety of experiences within the vast spectrum of the LGBTQIA+ world.

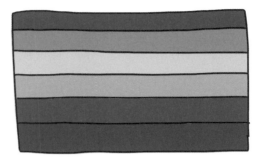

GAY PRIDE FLAG

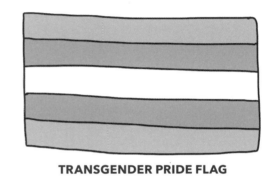

TRANSGENDER PRIDE FLAG

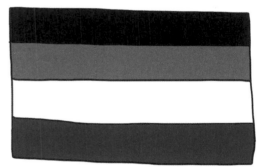

ASEXUALITY FLAG

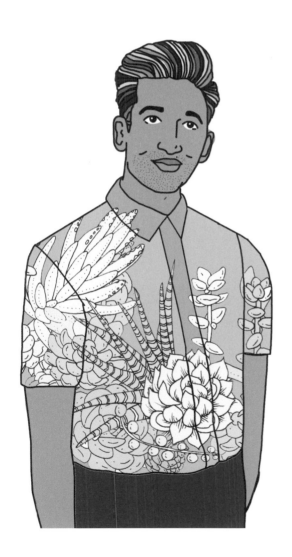

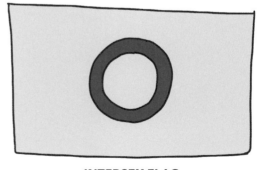

INTERSEX FLAG

The Dangers of the Coming Out Movement

If you are in an environment where you don't feel safe to be publicly in your gender or sexuality, **it's okay to protect yourself until it's safer.**

There can be a tendency to overemphasize the bravery of coming out, and see it as the golden key into the queer community. While it is a courageous act to be vulnerable with a larger community of friends and family, the act of coming out can lead to serious and dangerous consequences when made under societal pressure. There is often a narrative that it is only after coming out that we can be our fully complete, free, and honest selves. However, we can be complete in many ways. We each hold aspects of ourselves that are not public—trauma, secrets, fears, our bodies— which can come to light at any point.

It is incredibly important for the queer and trans-gender population to be visible, recognized, and respected. However, the faces of coming-out stories have predominantly been people with societal privilege. Queer and trans members of any community can potentially experience negative reactions or treatment when their gender or sexuality becomes public. However, queer people who experience other forms of marginalization because of race, class, and geographical location often face more extreme consequences of coming out, such as workplace discrimination, physical and sexual violence, harassment, online bullying, rejection from loved ones, and unstable housing.

If you know someone who has not yet publicly come out, be a support to them until they are ready to tell people. Don't pressure them or present coming out as the entry fee into the queer community. Too much value put on public visibility can risk harming individuals who do not have the privilege to guarantee their safety or stability once they come out.

Support them and be glad they trust you enough to let you into an incredibly personal experience.

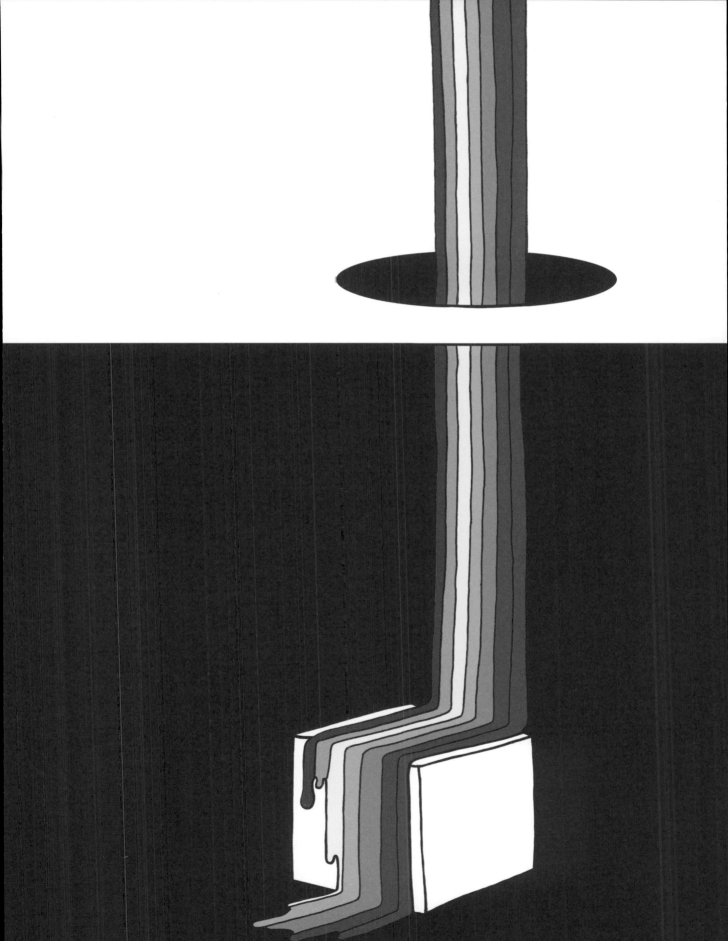

Matthew Shepard was a gay man who was beaten, tortured, and left to die on a rural fence post in Laramie, Wyoming, on October 6, 1998. He was found alive but succumbed to his injuries and died six days later.

His death brought attention to hate crimes against the LGBTQIA+ community, leading to the Matthew Shepard Act (officially known as the Matthew Shepard and James Byrd, Jr., Hate Crimes Prevention Act), which formally expanded the legislative definition of hate crimes to include crimes motivated by the victim's (perceived) gender, sexual orientation, gender identity, or disability.

There is debate about whether the killers' motivations were homophobia or the effects of drugs, and the reasons are still not totally known. Regardless, Shepard has remained an important figure in the fight for anti-hate crime law.

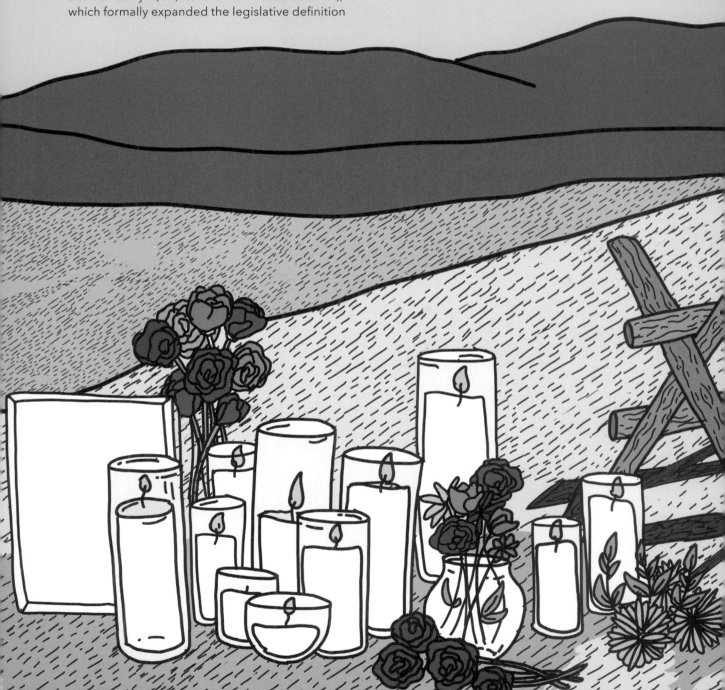

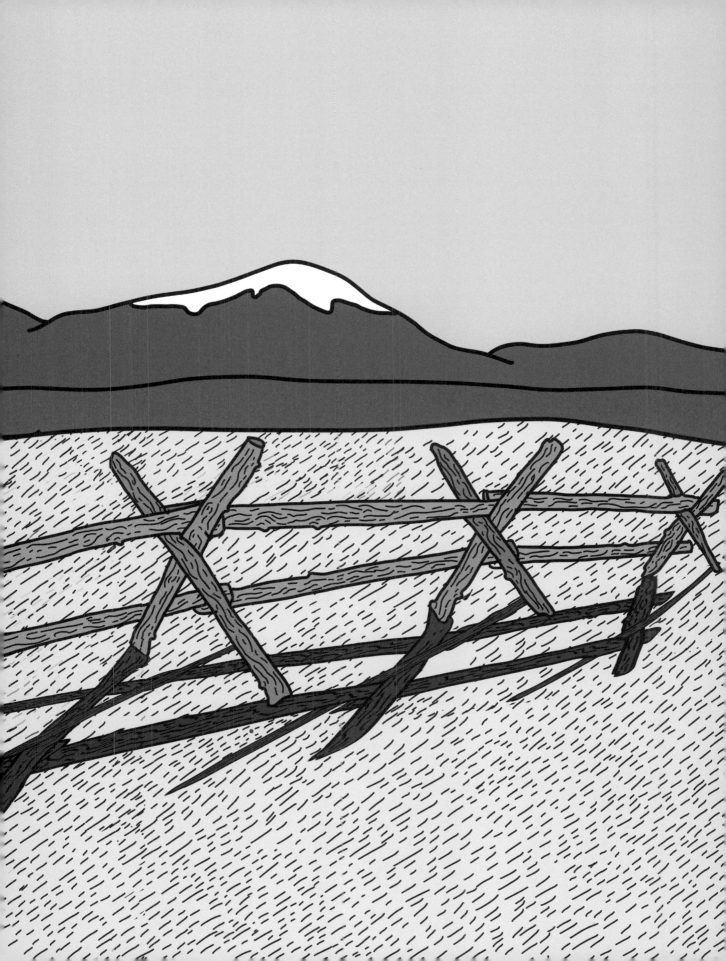

Advertising

Gender stereotypes are, and always have been, all over the advertising world. Some of these are obvious to those of us who have seen a television commercial or a magazine ad. A thin, bronzed white woman lying on a beach to advertise something totally unrelated, like beer. Young boys playing with Hot Wheels cars. Men driving sports cars. Women cleaning. Men ogling women. Buff men. Homemaker women. White people.

We recognize the overt ways that advertisements throw gender in our faces, but there are so many subliminal ways that ads can enforce roles of femininity and masculinity. They tell us that if we buy the right things, we'll be thinner, stronger, more beautiful, more handsome, richer, sexier, and smarter. We'll fit in with our own gender and/or be more attractive to the opposite gender. **They perpetuate unhealthy gender norms and can have huge, lasting effects on how we view gender roles.**

In 1911, the world came to the understanding that "sex sells." In a print ad for Woodbury Soap Company, an image of a woman being held by a man with the slogan "A Skin You Love to Touch" was published as the first major advertisement to objectify a woman. (What a milestone.) This ad implies that a woman's skin is primarily for a man's enjoyment, and only secondarily for her own enjoyment, and that she is meant to mold to his desires.

Seeing oneself portrayed as an object in mass media leads one to believe they are an object. All genders and body types can experience self-objectification, but it primarily affects women, who see themselves portrayed in media as unrealistic, dehumanized bodies used for a man's pleasure.

Bodies are used all the time in advertising to send specific, if subtle, messages to audiences. Even though objectifying women doesn't work very well when trying to sell products to women, it is effective in perpetuating gendered beauty standards. Similarly, handsome, muscular men in ads enforce the idea that in order to be manly or masculine, one must have a body that would require spending eight hours a day at the gym. Ads with larger body types in them are usually laced with shame and blame, causing internalized social discrimination against overweight people.

I haven't yet mentioned gender-non-conforming people in advertisements since historically there have been almost none. The only instances of gender bending have been men in dresses as a joke or men making fun of other men for being too sensitive. In the past couple of years, there has been an increase in the visibility of LGBTQIA+ people in commercials and print ads. Fashion has always played with androgyny, and lately there has been a resurgence of gender bending in the fashion world, which has made its way into print ads. It gets a bit confusing because many of the models who wear clothing typical of a different gender on the runway are cisgender. Remember, gender expression doesn't always mean gender identity (a man wearing feminine clothing can still identify as a man).

Non-binary models are still few and far between, and many of the opportunities to fill that androgynous niche are being filled by people who identify within the binary. Similar to how cisgender actors are hired for transgender roles in TV or movies, cisgender models are hired to play with androgyny, a job that should be given to non-binary models. People like Rain Dove (non-binary model), Andreja Pejic (trans model), Maria José (transfeminine model), Amandla Stenberg (non-binary actor and model), and Aaron Philip (disabled, trans, gender-fluid model) are pushing the boundaries of non-binary people in the spotlight and are hopefully some of the first in a long line of gender-variant people as the faces of media to come.

In 2017, Britain banned advertisements that promote damaging gender stereotypes. This includes objectifying or sexualizing women and girls, encouraging unhealthily thin bodies, or supporting a culture that mocks gender-non-conforming people.

There is still a lot of work to do in breaking advertisement stereotypes of bodies, race, and gender, but we can all work to be less influenced by what advertisers tell us we should be.

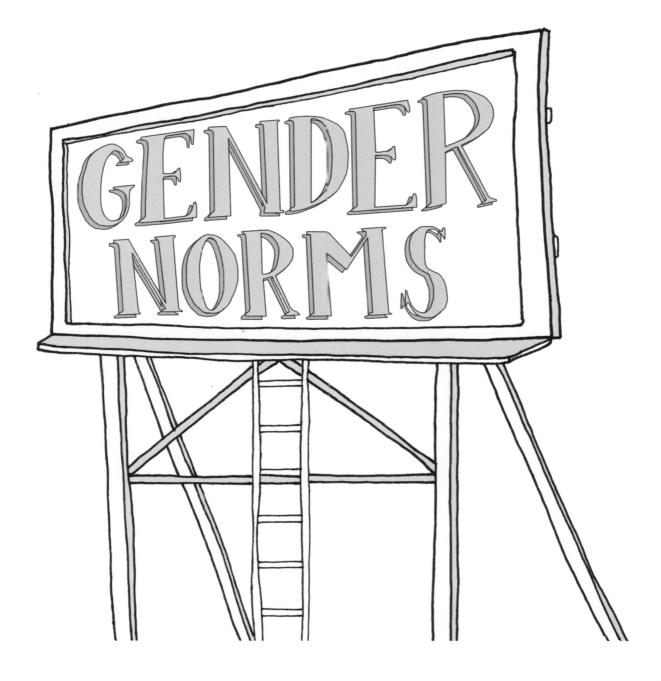

The Myth of Rosie the Riveter

We all know the iconic image of Rosie the Riveter: feminist hero of World War II and general symbol of feminism, right?

Well . . . maybe not so much.

The idea we currently have of this powerful image is mostly based on fiction. We think of the "We Can Do It" poster as a representation of female empowerment and feminism (and that friend who inevitably wears the jumpsuit and bandana for Halloween every year). But a message of empowerment wasn't the intention when the poster was originally issued. Although there were many recruitment posters at the time for female labor (with the men away at war), the "We Can Do It" poster wasn't one of them. Westinghouse Electric Corporation commissioned artist J. Howard Miller to paint a series of motivational posters to hang in its factories. The "We Can Do It" poster was one of many, and hung for only two weeks, an unmemorable blip. Miller didn't even name the woman in his poster "Rosie"; that name came from the next incarnation, painted by Norman Rockwell for the *Saturday Evening Post* in 1943. His version had a burly woman eating lunch, her foot smashing a copy of *Mein Kampf*. The name on her lunchbox? Rosie.

The "We Can Do It" image resurfaced in the 1980s during the fortieth anniversary of World War II and was quickly adopted as a feminist symbol of power, strength, and independence. Interestingly, some say Miller's image was chosen over Rockwell's, mostly because it wasn't copyrighted, and also didn't contain the Hitler reference, which made it easier to use in multiple contexts. It doesn't seem accidental that they chose the Rosie who was still clean and in makeup, a proper woman even in the factories.

Betty Reid Soskin, the country's oldest park ranger, works at the Rosie the Riveter museum in Richmond, California. Betty was alive during the time of Rosie's inception, and her memory of the reality behind the propaganda was not so rosy. She was a member of an all-Black, segregated women's factory union. When reflecting on the notion that the factories were a place of integrated unity among Black and white women, she says, "If you knew the sequence by which people were hired: first to be hired were the men who were too old to fight; second, the boys who were too young to be drafted; third, single white women; and when that pool was exhausted, married white women. And not until 1943, the first Black men were hired, as helpers and trainees only, to do the heavy lifting for the women they brought on board. And while there were some Black women who worked as laborers, sweeping the decks while other people worked, it wasn't until late in 1944, early in 1945, that Black women began to be trained as welders."

The myth of Rosie holds much optimism in her lore: inspiration, independence, strength, and a symbol of desegregation among female factory workers—even if it's a big ol' lie.

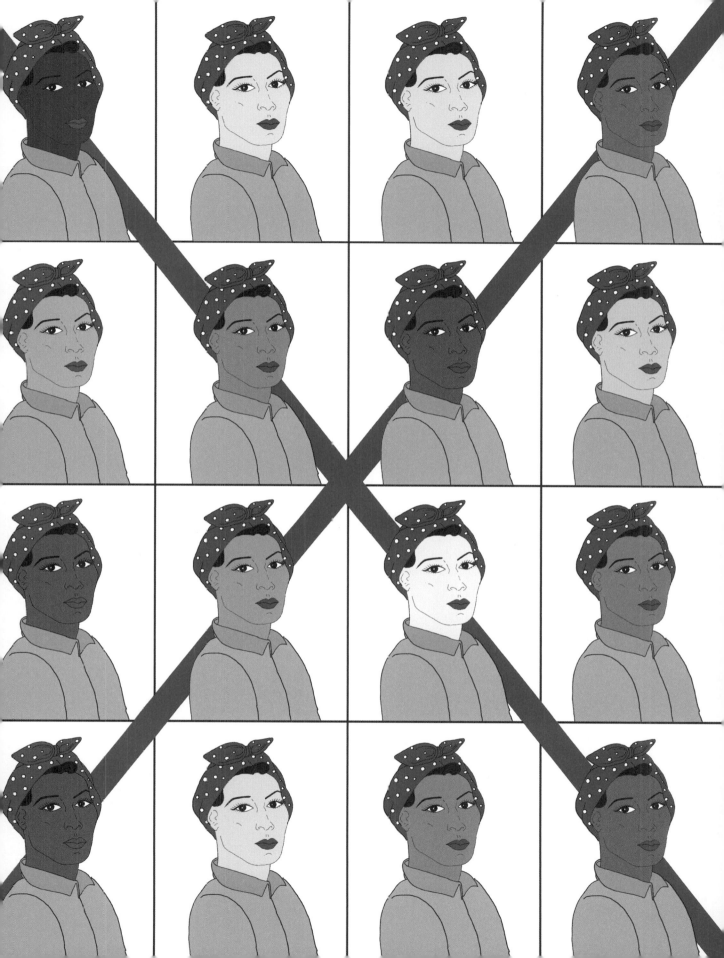

Spotlight on:
Hannah Gadsby

"To be rendered powerless does not destroy your humanity. Your resilience is your humanity. The only people who lose their humanity are those who believe they have the right to render another human being powerless. They are the weak. To yield and not break, that is incredible strength."

—HANNAH GADSBY

One of my favorite pieces of media in 2018 was Hannah Gadsby's stand-up special, *Nanette*. What I expected was an hour of her deadpan and sometimes dark humor, but what I got was so much more. It was a profound statement of anger and sadness, shame and honesty, and discussions of gender and mental illness—but not from behind the curtain of humor. She stepped right out in front of the curtain and tore it down.

Gadsby has worked as a comedian and writer for more than ten years, recently drawing international attention for *Nanette*. In this piece, there is a rawness of anger and truth that makes no attempt to comfort those watching. Gadsby is gender-non-conforming and queer, an identity that is discussed throughout the show as a center point of struggle, trauma, shame, pain, and anger throughout her life, one that has deeply shaped her as a person and a comedian. Much of the show is a dialogue about the potential damage that comedy and humor cause in the stories we tell about our experiences. She talks about the shame that accompanies internalized and public homophobia and how it morphed into the butt of her jokes, a point of humor rather than a revealing of pain. That damage didn't allow her to be vulnerable, or her story to be told in all its fullness and complexity.

She says, "I have built a career out of self-deprecating humor and I don't want to do that anymore. Do you understand what self-deprecation means when it comes from somebody who already exists in the margins? It's not humility, it's humiliation. I put myself down in order to speak, in order to seek permission to speak, and I simply will not do that anymore, not to myself or anybody who identifies with me. If that means that my comedy career is over, then so be it."

Nanette felt like an encapsulation of the moment we are both in and entering, where media allows marginalized people to have a platform from which to speak their truths. While this is far from perfect, far from complete, and far from wholly representative, it is certainly a brave and bold start.

Her final message to the audience emphasized connectedness, empathy, and learning. It's the same one I'm trying to spread in this book—to represent those stories less told, show the people who need to be seen, who need to see themselves represented to feel less alone, and to teach different perspectives to those who are open to learning.

Her closing message is this: "What I would have done to have heard a story like mine. Not for blame. Not for reputation, not for money, not for power. But to feel less alone. To feel connected. I want my story heard . . . I believe we could paint a better world if we learned how to see it from all perspectives, as many perspectives as we possibly could. Diversity is strength. Difference is a teacher. Fear difference, you learn nothing."

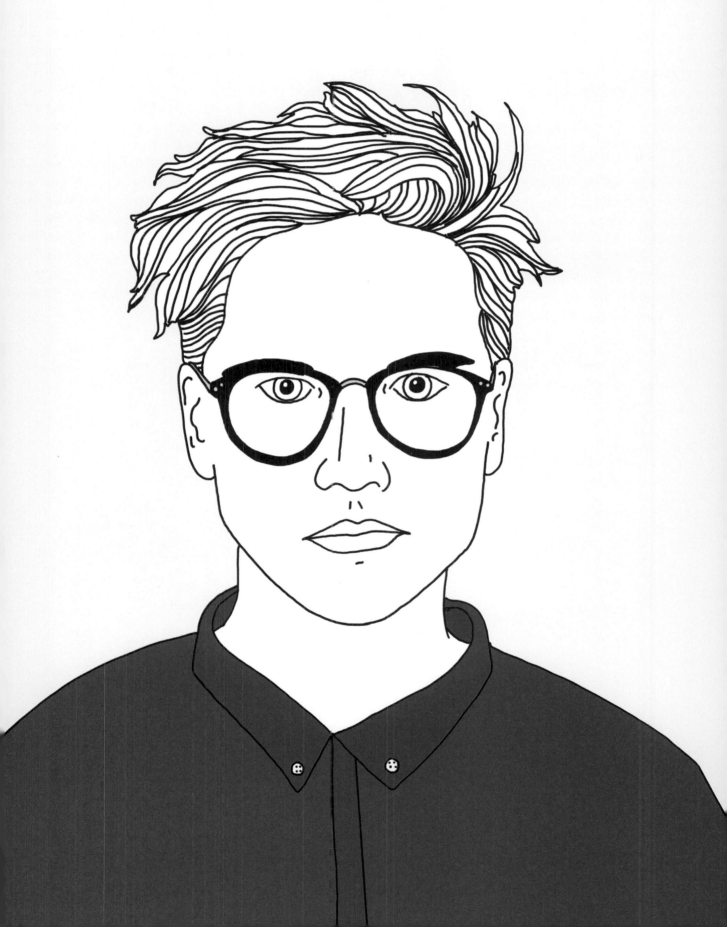

The Bechdel Test

QUESTION:

What do these movies have in common?

- *Harry Potter and the Deathly Hallows: Part II*
- *Lord of the Rings I, II, and III*
- *Ratatouille*
- *The Grand Budapest Hotel*
- *Avatar*
- *The Little Mermaid*
- *Citizen Kane*
- *The Social Network*
- *Finding Nemo*

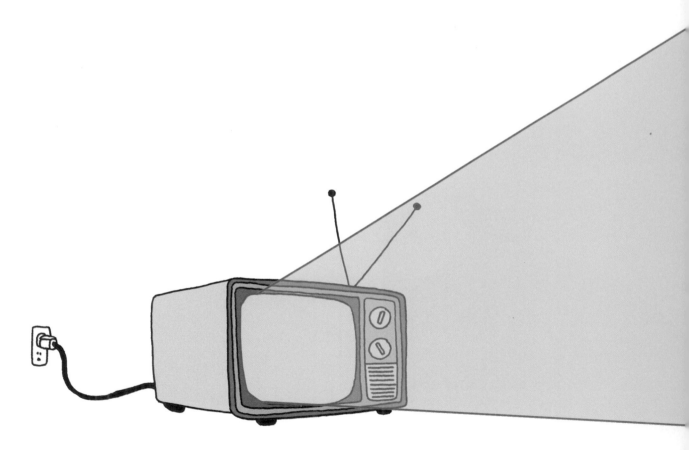

ANSWER:

None of them have two named female characters who speak to each other about something other than a man (or a male fish child in some cases).

The Bechdel test (or Bechdel-Wallace test) was originally created in 1985 as a joke by Alison Bechdel in her comic strip, *Dykes to Watch Out For*. Today the test is used by many film critics as a basic standard for feminism and female representation in films, video games, and television.

Obviously not all films would pass with these criteria, like certain nonfiction stories, films set in certain contexts (a male prison), or stories with essentially one character. This test also doesn't cover the full gamut of equal representation of gender by any means, nor does it measure the depth of non-male characters.

Only about 58 percent of films in the database at bechdeltest.com (going back to the nineteenth century) pass the test, so incomplete as the test may be, it still shows that equal gender representation in the history of films could have been much better.

Spotlight on:

Frank Ocean

Frank Ocean has become one of the most popular musicians of the last decade. Known for his evocative, vulnerable lyrics and inventive melding of musical genres, he began as a songwriter for big acts like Beyoncé, John Legend, and Brandy. He transformed into a solo artist around 2011 with the release of his first mixtape, *Nostalgia, Ultra*.

Before debuting his first full-length album, *Channel Orange*, in 2012, Ocean penned an open letter on Tumblr revealing that he'd been in love with a man. This honest and stripped-down announcement is the only explicit comment he's made about his sexuality, and even in the letter he didn't label himself with any sexual identity.

While queerness is not at the center of Ocean's music and career, it certainly is an identity that's woven throughout his music in honest and thoughtful ways. Many songs deal with first loves, unrequited love, and unpacking the intricacies of intimacy. Ocean is not a loud shouter of queerness like Freddie Mercury or Boy George; he allows for and encourages ambiguity in his lyrical references and refuses to label himself.

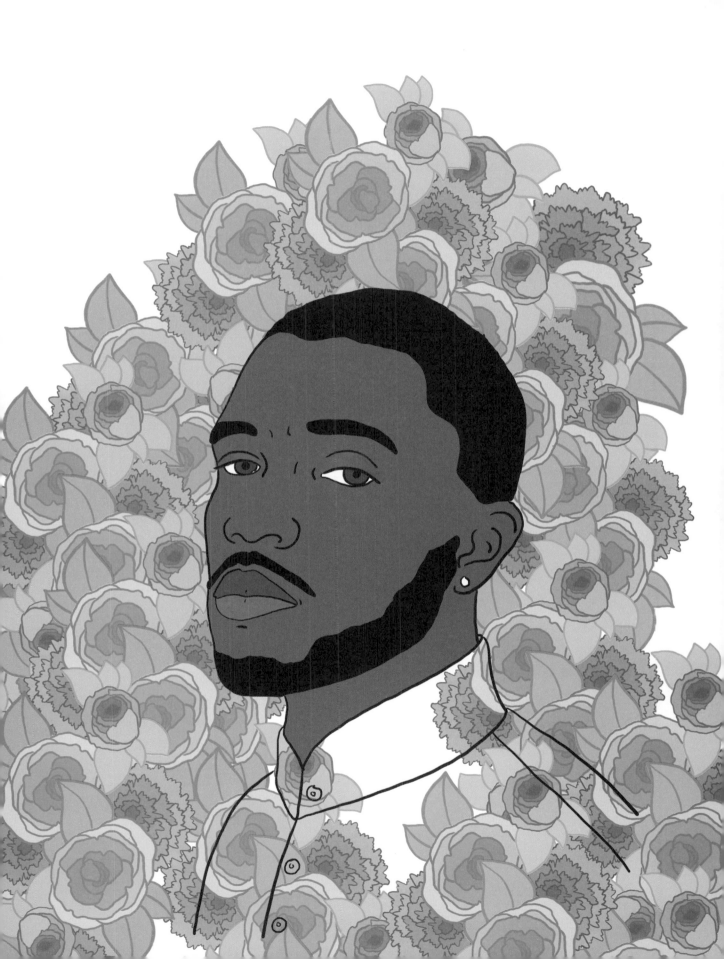

What Most Aligns with or Describes Your Gender in This Moment?

So much of gender expression and identity is body-based—our physical form, clothing, makeup, social groups, names, and how we carry ourselves. I was curious to know if people felt connected to things outside of themselves as representative of their gender, so I asked strangers to submit their answers to this question.

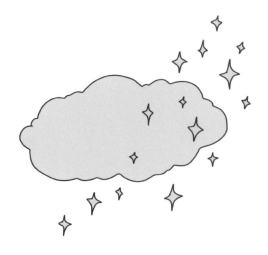

Name: Sequoyah
Age: 6
Gender identity: I don't really know my gender yet. I'm both of the famous genders: boys and girls.
What most aligns with or describes your gender in this moment? A wish.

Name: Ben
Age: 53
Gender identity: FTM (female-to-male)
What most aligns with or describes your gender in this moment? My California driver's license with my bearded face, birth name, and "F" gender marker.

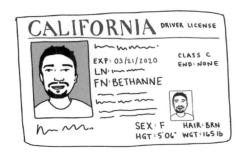

Name: Ike
Age: 21
Gender identity: Man
What most aligns with or describes your gender in this moment? A "women's" T-shirt inside my closet. A few months ago, I bought this loose yellow cropped shirt. I cut the sleeves and painted red flames on the lower part (it kinda looks like the yellow car in the movie *Kill Bill*). Since then it has stayed inside my wardrobe. I'm a very hairy guy, and have been heteronormative my entire life, both in the way I behave and in the relationships I have. A couple years

ago I got really depressed and since then, started to question everything, including my sexuality and gender. I still don't know what I identify as (gender-wise) and have been trying new stuff from different clothes to breaking my boxed male behaviors. But I still don't have the courage to wear the yellow cropped T-shirt that lives in my closet.

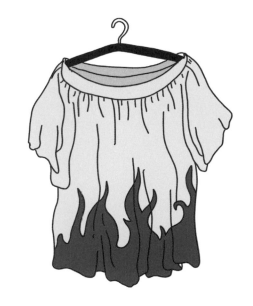

Name: Alyson
Age: 32
Gender identity: Cisgender female who is gender non-conformist
What most aligns with or describes your gender in this moment? My gender is a road bike—specifically my midnight blue Giant Peloton with drop handle-bars. I've chosen this as a disabled person. My bike gives me so much more comfort and freedom than painful, weight-bearing walking alone or carrying anything; it's almost like a form of mobility device. I'm here, I'm queer, and my chronic pain is severe! It also makes me androgynous. Anyone on a bike is just a cyclist (especially in my comfortable and sexy spandex kits). I love the anonymous and androgynous appearance cycling gives me.

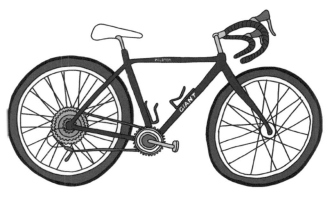

Name: Anonymous
Age: 21
Gender identity: Male
What most aligns with or describes your gender in this moment? My denim jacket! It was my mom's in the '90s and she gave it to me when I was in high school. It's my favorite article of clothing. I have cool pins and patches on it. I appreciate that my mom gave it to me—I often credit my mom with a lot of negativity in my life, especially because of her angry, resentful response when I came out as a gay trans man. But this jacket feels like an important symbol of her love for me, which I hope is growing as she progresses in her acceptance of me. Basically, my jacket symbolizes a few of the most important influences on my life, identity, and future—my mom, my community and my community's history, and also myself, in the way that I have adorned the jacket and made it my own. I feel like my jacket is just . . . me, my gender, my gay/trans/Latino self, represented in one (stylish, timeless) piece of clothing.

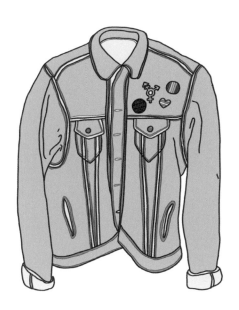

Name: Aron
Age: 18
Gender identity: Trans male
What most aligns with or describes your gender in this moment? My gender in this moment feels like a long, long drive that I am stuck in the middle of, and the scenery is beautiful, and I am not upset at the journey, but I have been in this car too long to care anymore, and my clothes don't fit right, and my back aches, and the next stop isn't for seventy-three more miles and it feels like I won't make it there before dark.

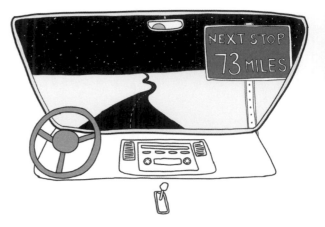

Name: Victoria
Age: 30
Gender identity: Femme
What most aligns with or describes your gender in this moment? I wear this head scarf most days since becoming a parent. Giving birth has changed and in some ways broken my body. Which clothes fit me changes daily. My hair is a mess as I run my broken body, mood disorder, and medically complex child to appointments. This simple head scarf always fits, makes me feel queer and femme and tough. Maybe even visible.

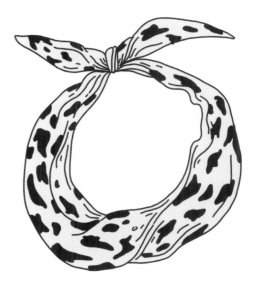

Name: Jade
Age: 20
Gender identity: Non-binary trans boy
What most aligns with or describes your gender in this moment? A pair of small clip-on rose earrings that used to belong to my lola. After realizing I identified as trans, shifting my presentation to be more masculine felt really affirming and good. But I still have an attachment to some traditionally "feminine" items, like my lola's earrings. She was a really special person to me and taught me that the spiritual element of life is one without contradiction, one that always rebalances itself. When I wear these earrings, I feel the radiant calm and love that she provided when she was alive, and wearing them with super-short hair and boy clothes makes me feel 100 percent like my mischievous queer self. Even if my lola wouldn't have fully understood my identity, I know she would have loved that I have finally learned to be happy in who I am. Although the journey is hard, I'm so glad that she is still with me.

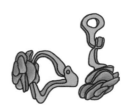

Name: AC
Age: 11
Gender identity: Non-binary/agender
What most aligns with or describes your gender in this moment? I have chosen my headphones/earbuds, mainly because music works as a coping mechanism for me. Whenever I feel dysphoric or sad for some reason, I can listen to music and it reminds me that everything will be okay again.

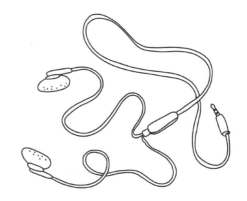

Name: Casy
Age: 17
Gender identity: Non-binary
What most aligns with or describes your gender in this moment? My hair. I always had my parents and grandparents decide what to do with my hair. When I made a decision to shave my head for a charity fundraiser event called St. Baldricks, I not only felt liberated by the experience, but I finally felt free to do what I wanted with my hair. It was the first amount of control I had had over my appearance in my life and it still plays a big part in my identity.

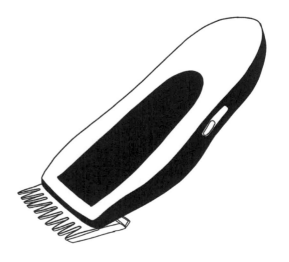

Name: Rowena
Age: 25
Gender identity: Female
What most aligns with or describes your gender in this moment? Things that make me feel feminine are things that make me feel strong and beautiful. Shaving my head made me feel just like this, even though I think a lot of women (and men/non-binary peeps) would see their hair as their source of beauty. It felt so empowering, cool, sexy, and feminine to shave all my hair off. I always find women with shaved heads alluring and intriguing, there's nothing more interesting than someone subverting beauty standards. Therefore, my lack of hair is this thing that best aligns with my own gender identity. :)

Name: Bill
Age: 3
Gender identity: A knight
What most aligns with or describes your gender in this moment? I picked a knight because I wish I was a knight. I'm brave and strong, but I don't eat my carrots.

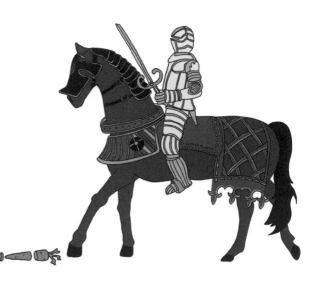

Name: Mandi
Age: 32
Gender identity: Femme tomboy
What most aligns with or describes your gender in this moment? A baseball cap. I stole it from my best friend/crush when I was thirteen. I was deep into my teenage tomboy phase and wore it everywhere, along with baggy track pants, a too-big T-shirt, and an extra-large hoodie. I prided myself on breaking out of gender expectations: I wore boxers until I was eleven, refused to wear makeup and tank tops, and my favorite weekend activity was going to the junkyard with my dad, a mechanic. Fast-forward twenty years, during which I've come to appreciate tight jeans and fitted tees (though I stand firm on my discomfort with makeup), and I'm reevaluating how I present myself to the world. For the past eight months, I've had a desire to reclaim my tomboyishness, and I've been thinking about buying a new baseball cap—I still only own the one from my teens. So, this grungy old hat has become a symbol of who I truly am: a creative and curious tinkerer who is still growing.

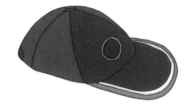

Name: Kelly
Age: 36
Gender identity: Female
What most aligns with or describes your gender in this moment? My ratty old (broken) nursing bra. Prior to having my only son (who will be two in two days) I struggled for years to get pregnant. After nursing for almost twenty-three months, I am excited for my freedom but also feeling big feelings about these parts of my body which have a different function now. The ending of nursing lined up with a second pregnancy loss. I am at an apex in my life, wondering if I love the freedom of my body over trying to house another life again. I identify as a woman and a mom but also as someone with profound sadness over loss and infertility.

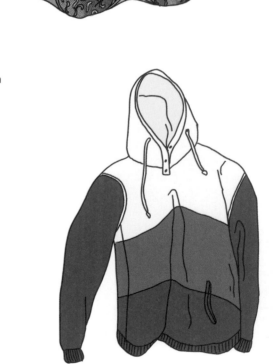

Name: Mako
Age: 17
Gender identity: Non-binary
What most aligns with or describes your gender in this moment? I have chosen oversized sweaters, because they let me be comfortable and their excess fabric makes my shape less defined.

Name: Lindsay
Age: 21
Gender: Agender
What most aligns with or describes your gender in this moment? My gender is some indistinguishable embryo sitting in a museum or laboratory. Most embryos look the same at the beginning, regardless of whether they'll develop into a fish or a mammal or reptile or bird or other evolved life form. It's only as they develop specific organs that they can be differentiated from this starting plan, the blueprint of a wallaby or a falcon or a dolphin. My gender is this baseline embryo sitting on a shelf in a jar of ethanol—it's not growing, changing, or developing. It never was and never will be, but I still appreciate that there are wallabies and falcons and dolphins in the world.

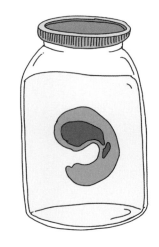

Name: Will
Age: 30
Gender identity: Trans man, transmasculine, and also transfemme these days with my beard and skirts. Definitely non-binary.
What most aligns with or describes your gender in this moment? My hairy boobs! I never see representation of folks on testosterone who choose not to get top surgery. I like that they are so hairy. I want to chestfeed my babies some day and I thought it would be this weird gross thing for them to suck on but then I got over it. Now I love them. They feel weird and whimsical, just like me.

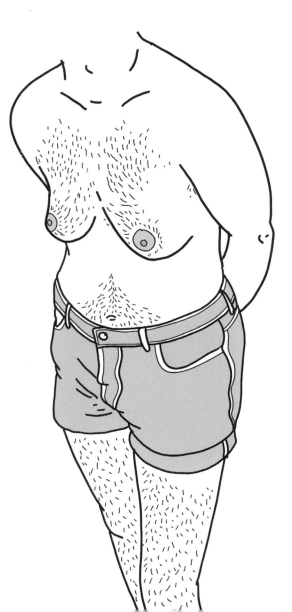

Name: Cassy
Age: 30
Gender identity: Confident enigmatic sparkly boyband (gender non-conforming/genderqueer)
What most aligns with or describes your gender in this moment? At this exact moment, I think my gender is best captured by imagining Jonathan Van Ness and Tan France on a best friend date riding horses together in a meadow overlooking gorgeous mountains filled with aspen trees talking about Xena the Warrior Princess.

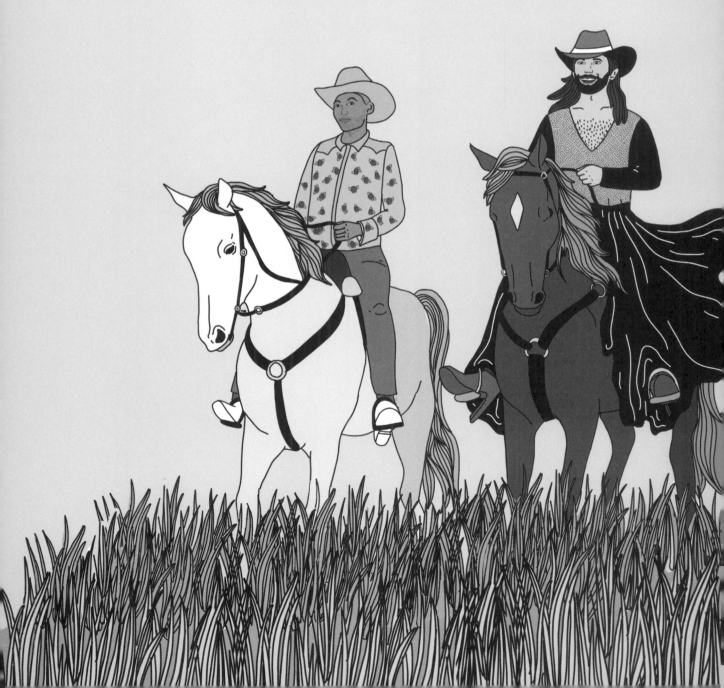

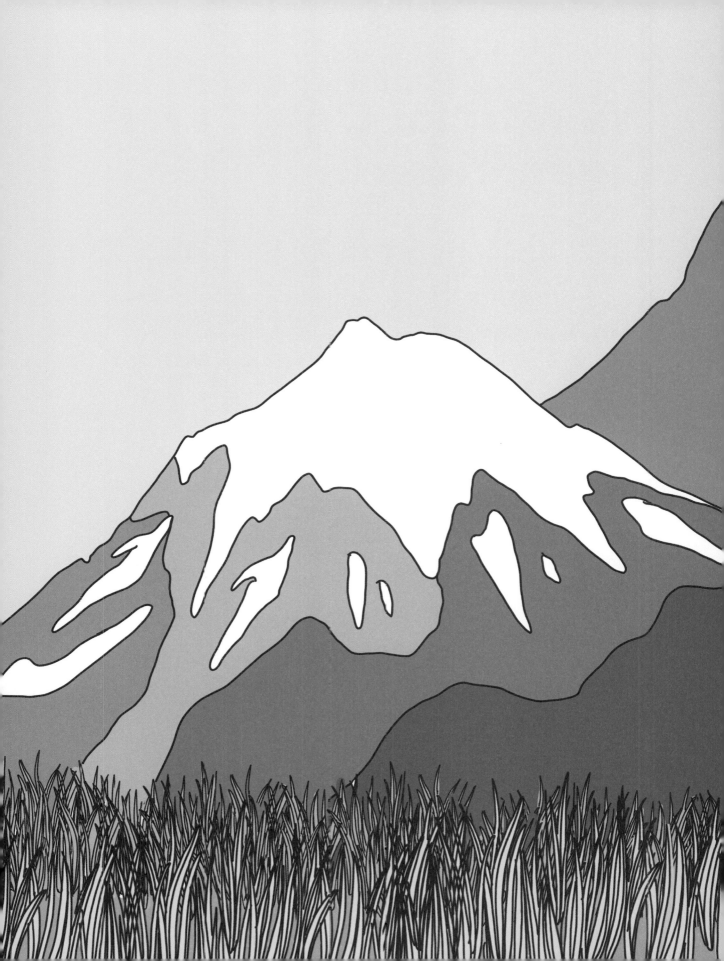

We Are Not Only Our Categories

Much of this book focuses on defining terms, identities, and categorizations that break down groupings of gender, sexuality, and identity into smaller units. It's useful to have this language when introducing concepts, explaining unfamiliar experiences to those outside of yourself, and connecting with people who share that experience. Sometimes, though, a million subcategories can feel just as divisive as two broad categories.

In having infinite identities and descriptors—particularly around gender and sexuality—we must also keep in mind that having a certain identity doesn't necessarily mean you must remain in that identity forever, or that you must adhere to all the unwritten rules that define that label. At the end of the day, we are unique and impossible to categorize.

Let's keep flexible and open, allowing for change within ourselves and others. Every change is valid in every stage.

All of us are shapeshifters.

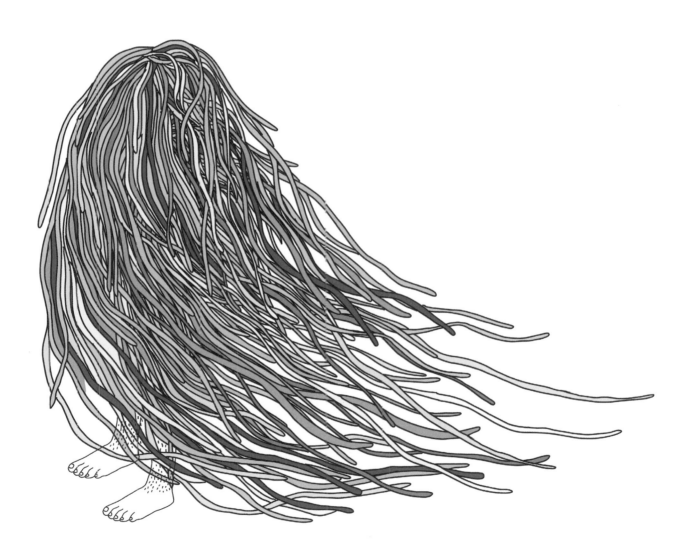

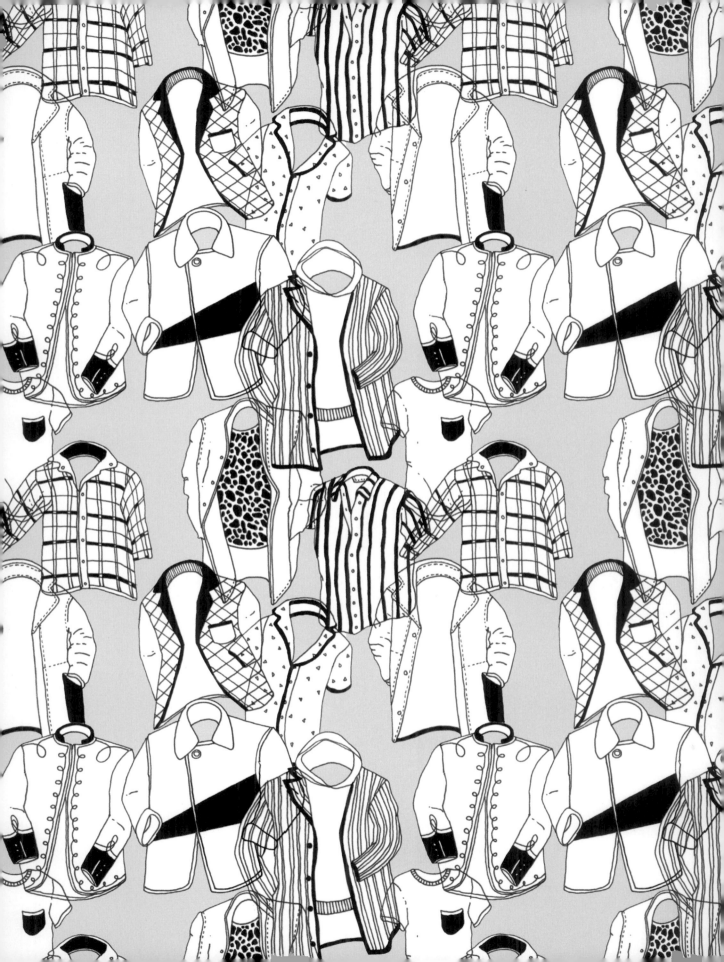

My Story

How Harry Styles Made Me the Boy I Am Today

Harry Styles transformed notions of my own gender, sexuality, body, and fashion.

In the summer of 2017, I was playing around with creating patterns for wallpaper or fabric and really wanted to do a design featuring highly patterned menswear. After some searching for reference images, I found the holy grail of fun-to-draw clothing: Harry Styles's wardrobe. I didn't really know of him before—I'm of the Backstreet Boys era. But seeing his long hair swooped to one side, flamboyant button-up shirts (unbuttoned more often than not), and shiny shimmery floral suits, I felt so envious and attracted to his confident gender play (and I have a deep love of pretty boys, which helps). There is something so queer about his style—so wildly different from mine—but it would ultimately become a hugely important influence on my own gender.

At the time I discovered Harry, I thought of my gender as a piece of moss, just hanging out with no desire to have a body, clinging to a rock and enjoying a nice view of the woods indefinitely. Unnoticed and unimportant (I'm not going to pretend my self-esteem was high). Since I am, most unfortunately, a human, I identified as female, but rather apathetically. I had been queer-identified for about five years and was in the ongoing process of figuring out what external gender expression matched with my internal gender identity, both ambiguous unknowns at the time. I acquired some femme clothes and jewelry to explore one of the many sides of the expression spectrum after many years of dressing relatively gender-neutral or masculine of center. Let's just say the femme trial was a short-lived, failed experiment. Yikes.

I had always had a strong sense of body dysmorphia, which for a long time I was unaware was related to gender or sexuality. In this early Harry Styles era, it manifested as wearing oversized shirts to hide my chest, a hat to cover up my weird partially bleached mullet (indecisively trying both short hair and long, blond and brown at the same time), and ratty cut-off shorts that hung off my ass. A far cry from a shimmery floral suit.

I was obsessed with living vicariously through Harry Styles as a well-dressed boy in a boy-ish body. It led me to believe maybe I was a . . . boy . . . of some sort? (A real a-ha moment.) This was not such a massive leap from my version of genderqueer, but the mental shift to seeing myself as a boy ("she-boy" as I liked to say at the time) was the first time I felt a click of accuracy between my body and my identity.

My fashion crush became a recurring visitor in both my waking and dream lives, and I decided I needed to write him a letter, explaining how he positively (and confusingly) influenced my existential crisis so heavily. At the time, I was visiting my parents' house for a month. There was a three-hour time difference, it was very hot, and the guest bed was less comfy than I would have liked. I would unsuccessfully attempt to sleep for a while, give up, and then stay up for hours crafting this letter. What started as a letter to an unreachable celebrity morphed into a journal of sorts, a conversation with myself, working out the resulting emotional and mental twists and turns sparked by this gender envy.

What I didn't anticipate was how desire and gender could collide with sexuality in an extremely confusing way. I identify as asexual. This means many things to many people, and like all sexualities, it has endless variations within itself, as well as the potential to morph over time. Even though I've identified with this term for quite some time, I still oscillate between feeling that it's a superpower and thinking I'm broken or deficient. I fear people will be disinterested in pursuing me before even knowing me because of the wide range of assumptions tied to that identity, a sense of "why bother?" If you don't have a good working relationship with the body you inhabit, and in fact deeply resent it, it makes the already difficult challenge of determining a gender identity that feels good in your body even harder. I truly wasn't sure what aspects of this confusion were the desire to be with someone (romantically or physically), be like someone, or to be liked by someone. I think all three.

I had considered getting top surgery (double mastectomy) for quite some time to feel more comfortable in my otherwise lanky boyish body (and have since gotten it), but suddenly I had a fearful wonder: would changing my body to reflect a gender identity more similar to someone I desire make me less desirable to them (and a theoretically larger population)? I have dated only women and non-binary people, so a boy-crush is somewhat of a foreign territory. If I am a queer she-boy with half of a "female body" and half of a "boy body," would boys who are straight be attracted to my boy body? Or would gay boys be attracted to my female body? And does asexuality make all of that null and void?

Objectively, I would argue that what matters most is what makes you most comfortable in your body. Personally, it felt scary to envision such a permanent change to the body I had lived in for twenty-nine years, especially when it could make me feel even

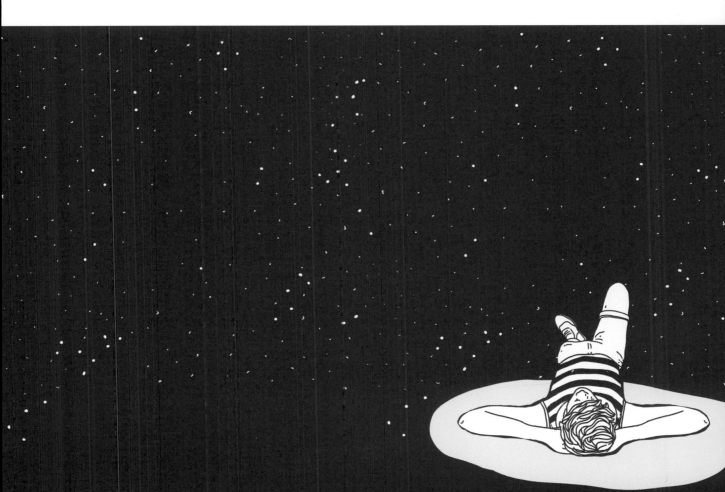

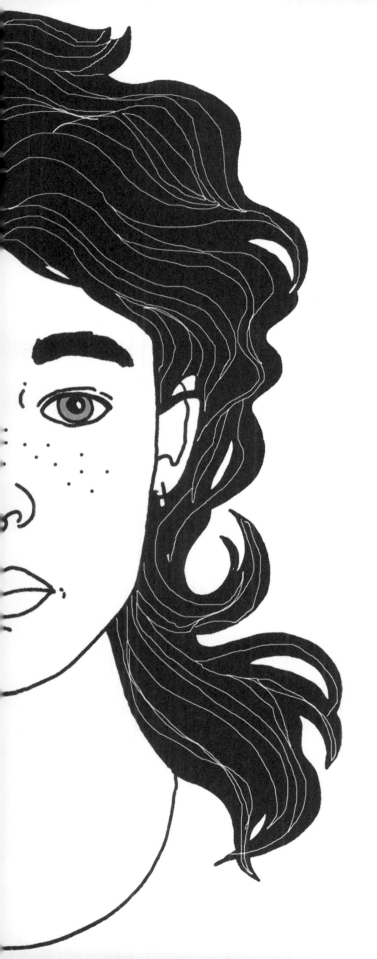

more isolated in my body experience. I was changing from an identifiable (albeit uncomfortable) body to an amalgamation of bodies. It was a scary thought from a medical standpoint for sure, but in me also rose a deep fear of being a chimera. A Frankenstein's monster of bodies.

During this time, Harry Styles was still a frequent visitor in my unconscious world. Yeah, I know, I know, I know that sounds creepy, but a sleeping brain does what it wants. Not my fault. We had a dynamic that was intensely parallel to the questions he symbolized in my waking life. My unconscious self was grappling with the exact same questions I was processing in my letter writing. Much of our interaction was me feeling ashamed of my queerness, my sexuality, and my body. We had a good time together, laughed and talked easily, but I consistently assumed I would never be viewed as a romantic prospect for him because I was too queer, too androgynous, too confusing, and that goddamn mullet was too ugly (it really, really was). We platonically shared a bed, and in the morning, all I had to offer were two tiny glasses of orange juice and a giant bowl of Cheetos—a definite selling point in my opinion.

There was a heartbreaking moment in one dream in which I put together a beautiful package of drawings with a thoughtful and vulnerable letter for him, the same one that I had been working on for weeks in waking life. It was a beautiful gift that I was really proud of, and it perfectly represented traits of my core self: gentle assertiveness, me as a giver of small handmade things and unexpected romantic gestures for such a generally disgruntled person. He had implied that he was going on a first date with someone that night who was a very straight, femme, glamorous, conventionally attractive woman and as I was preparing to hand the package to him, he said, "If I fall in love with her tonight, do you still want me to have this?" The honest answer was "No." That moment of understanding was a clear but sad fulfillment of my fear of rejection. It seemed that one date with someone stereotypically attractive in the gender norms that I do not adhere to was enough to prove to him that regardless of a fun, interesting, budding relationship, my intersection of identities was in and of itself a dealbreaker.

I have learned through this strange process that someone's gender presentation doesn't automatically reveal other facets of their identity. My collection of labels (asexual + genderqueer + lover of pretty boys + trans-questioning + deeply anxious) wasn't adding up to create much confidence—which shows how limiting labels can be, and how expansive anxiety can be. The equation doesn't matter much, since all of those terms are so tangled up with an individual's personality. My assumption of Harry's gender as a reflection of desire is unfair; just because he looks like a boy doesn't necessarily mean he identifies as one and/or wouldn't be into a boy-ish person. These assumptions of mine are as dangerous and incorrect as my fear of him (or anyone) shrinking my complexity into a simple assumption made from the clothing I wear.

I am in a different place now because of this process. I'm in a better and more confident place (or at least working on it). I got top surgery, I have much nicer short hair, and yet all the fears and points of confusion elicited during this time are still part of my life. I feel confused about my sexuality and I continue to see boys around and covet their bodies and sharp jawlines and don't quite feel like I'll ever fully understand how to be in my body. I want Harry Styles to think I'm great, to let me draw his closet, and date me even if I have no boobs. But until then, I want to give him a big thank-you.

Harry, I'm sorry this was such an intense introduction, but here's the letter from that beautiful package I was never able to give you:

Hi, my name is Iris—nice to meet you, Harry.

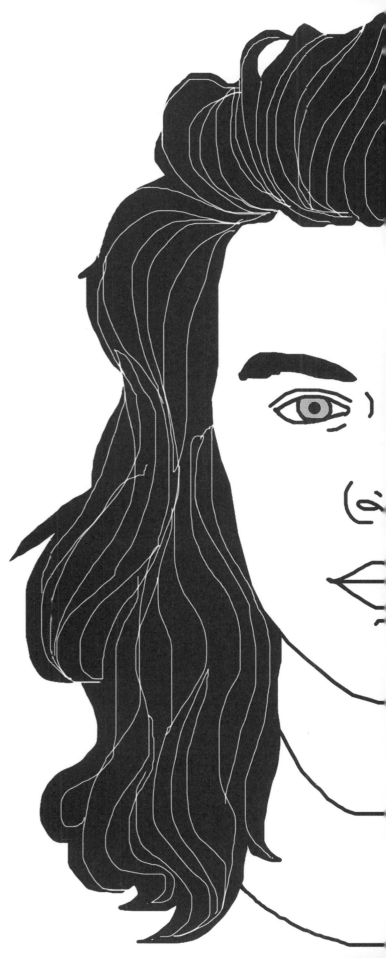

Ungendering and Desexualizing a Body

Eating Disorders

I've had anorexia since 2006, and I will likely always have it to some degree. It has ebbed and flowed in severity over time, from going vegetarian, to being told to leave college, to almost dying, to attending residential treatment, to now, where periods of distress lead to periods of not eating much. Even though it's been a decade since my illness was at its most severe and I live a healthy life now, my body is still permanently affected by the disorder, and I am reminded often of my history. Now more than ever, I can see the conflicting cultural assumptions of gender, sexuality, femininity, race, class, and mental illness at play within my own body.

Our bodies and genders are inextricably entangled, and the way people read our bodies informs their idea of our gender. It's difficult to divorce our understanding of our bodies from the gender binary, as we tend to see certain physical attributes as being more feminine or masculine.

My anorexia developed alongside my body when I was a teenager: I developed breasts and started my period earlier than most of my peers. I hated it. I did not want an adult female body, a feeling I'm sure many middle schoolers share. My illness crept in as I began to feel more and more uncomfortable with a body that was supposed to be sexual. I essentially stopped physically and emotionally developing at age seventeen. My period stopped for six years, I had early stages of osteoporosis, no hormonal hunger signals, and limited social interactions. While it was devastatingly shameful to be so visibly ill at my worst point (weighing only ninety pounds at 5'7"), there was safety in being sexually invisible and inhabiting a genderless, almost non-human body. Somewhere deep, deep down, my sixteen-year-old self knew something about my gender that I wouldn't fully recognize for a long time.

Now when I relapse, it's much more conscious—I don't mean it's consciously chosen (no one chooses to have an eating disorder)—but I am aware that being a string bean (very thin) allows me to be closer to the gender I align with. Having a lanky boy body with fewer curves helps me deal with the dysphoria of being genderqueer. I experience this from a position of privilege in which I do not experience fat phobia in combination with a genderqueer presentation. Thinness makes me feel less feminine, not more, despite the overwhelming marketing that thinness in people AFAB means achieving an ideal standard of femininity.

I also recently processed an aspect of my illness that I was always too ashamed of and confused by to understand: Being thin meant having a prominent jawline. This was one of the very first things that instigated my desire to look different. It wasn't even about the string bean at that point, just about the jaw. Now that I am in the process of moving toward embodying my version of "boy," I realize that I still consider a strong jaw to be conspicuously masculine and something I covet in others.

I still resent my illness for robbing me of my late teens and early twenties. And yet, I'm grateful that I developed such a strong system of self-preservation in the face of things that felt dangerous: being sexualized, being female, being at parties, being expected to abide by social norms. I fully bypassed that world to the detriment of many other things—but that time granted me a unique opportunity to be self-aware and exist outside the pressure cooker of adolescence.

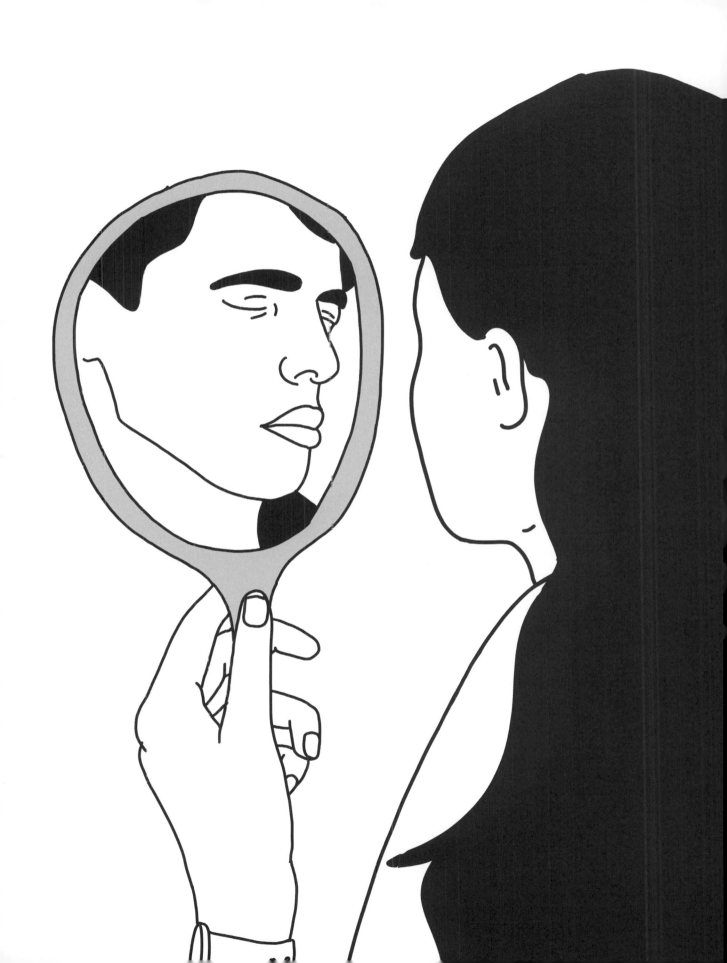

Surgery Journey
Grieving a Living Body

In three weeks, I am scheduled to have both of my breasts removed.

At the time of this writing, I have lived in this body for twenty-nine years, and while I am uncomfortable with how it conveys my gender, I will also mourn what I lose by changing my body permanently through surgery. I wish someone had told me about the grief that comes along with correcting gender dysphoria. How it is possible to simultaneously experience the sadness of loss of self, and the joy of reaching a truer self through that loss.

Sadness is okay, and sadness doesn't indicate it's a wrong choice.

It's hard to parse out the elements of grief as I say goodbye to a physical and emotional part of myself—something that has literally been attached to me for all this time. Something my body made from itself. Something that has represented so much struggle for so long. A decision that means saying goodbye to my previous genders.

I am voluntarily ridding myself of something that is objectively valued as a sign of beauty and replacing it with visible scars of my decision. My internalized transphobia speaks loudly as I fear that I am trading a standard of beauty for a standard of stigma. I know I will be loved well by those people who don't care about some fatty tissue, and I might inspire some people to love people who look like me, but I have to convince my emotional self of that as well. It's pretty ironic that altering my body to facilitate self-confidence creates a new realm of self-consciousness.

I feel grateful I have the ability and safety to do this, but I feel angry that I have to. That I have to get surgery to wear a T-shirt in the world without upset. That I have to prove to the government that I am "trans enough" or in enough emotional pain to qualify for surgery. That I have to fear for my safety and my future health care because of this. That the current president of the United States has banned the word *transgender* from use by the CDC.

I want people to know that it's okay to feel angry and scared and sad about saying goodbye to some of yourself and still know that it's the right thing to do.

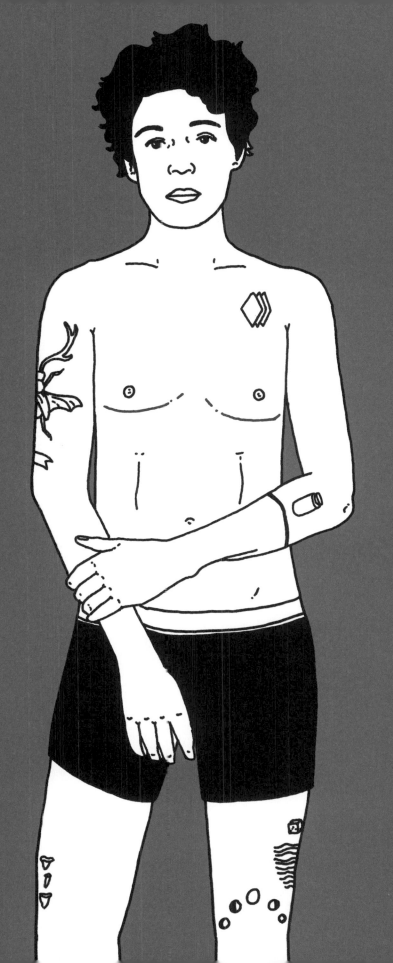

Surgery Journey Week Two:

Ritual

JUNE 3, 2018

I haven't felt very confident in the past two weeks; I've felt tired and disheveled and sore and gross. But last night I laid on the kitchen table while a friend poured hot water over my dirty dirty soapy hair, washing it for the first time since surgery. It felt like a baptism into my new self, a cleansing of worry and doubt. I put on a shirt afterward and finally knew for the first time that it was the right decision, even with all the emotional complexities that still exist.

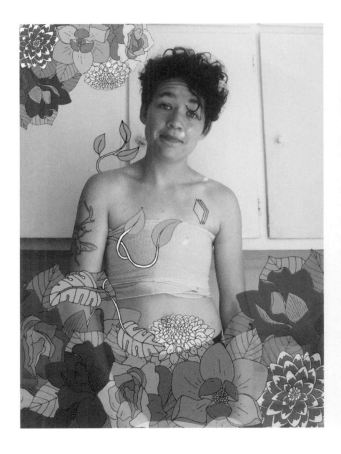

Surgery Journey Week Three:

First Skin

JUNE 11, 2018

At every appointment I've had and every time someone has needed to touch my chest after surgery, I have fainted or become wildly nauseous. I have been so overwhelmed by the sensation of patchy numbness, tingling, scarring, and touch in a place that is totally new to my recomposed body. When the large Ace wrap came off, I hunched all day, so the fabric of my shirt wouldn't touch my skin. My shoulders hurt so much from being hunched over for twenty-one days.

I took a shower for the first time earlier this week. I stepped into the tub with my eyes closed, still not ready to see the scars, and the moment water hit my back I became paralyzed in a half-crumpled sob. I kept my eyes closed for the entire time I was showering, while being helped around in my darkness. After stepping out of the shower, I kept my eyes shut until I was all bandaged up, so when I opened them, I couldn't see the scars.

It's three weeks post-surgery today, and last night I looked at the bottom incisions for the first time (not the nipple grafts, cuz that's too intense for right now). It was really okay. I got to secretly peel off some of the purple binding glue, a small reward for feeling brave. The body is amazing in its ability to heal, recover, and remake itself anew. I wore a T-shirt today for the first time into the world. It's light purple and flat against my front. I can finally stand up straight. My mom helped me try on a jumpsuit with my eyes closed. It fit like a perfect flat, baggy sack.

I am experiencing a lot of firsts. First touch, first skin, first shower, first T-shirt, first time standing upright. This is an overwhelming process, even as I step into it a little more each day. I relate to myself in a different way, afraid yet embracing. Realizing I don't need to be any gender other than whatever the hell I am. I don't need to be trans, non-binary, or any title at all. I'll stick with being a rectangle she-boy who loves Harry Styles and stripes. It really doesn't (and shouldn't) matter to me or anyone else that I am some amorphous being. Because it's all made up by us humans to begin with.

And so, the process continues.

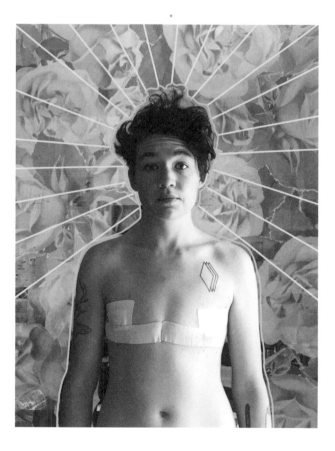

Surgery Journey Week Four:

Home

JUNE 18, 2018

It's been easy this week.

I don't have many profound thoughts other than feeling more at home in my body. I can touch and look at my incisions, which are turning pink and smooth. Every day they change, and every day I am getting used to the previous day and being surprised by the next. I got scared that they placed the nipples too far apart (in what feels like my armpits). But apparently they are just like that on boy people. I learned that under every boob is a pec muscle that can twitch and move. I was afraid of this change, afraid of this process, afraid of regret, afraid it would hurt and look ugly—afraid in general. But now I feel good.

I'm making another big change in a week: after five and a half years in California, I'm moving home to North Carolina. It feels like a wave of transition as I move back to my home place with my home self. I will feel all of these feelings while driving away from California and settling into my new old place, but I have been slowly planning both transitions for years and will slowly feel more and more sure about them with every passing week. When you move, like it or not, you take you with you—at least that feels good.

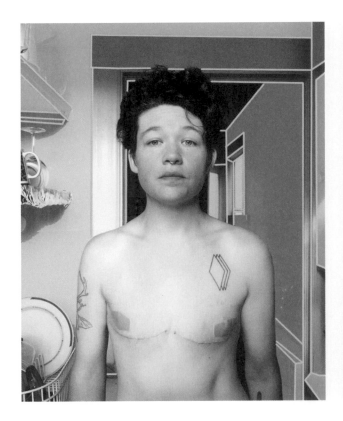

Surgery Journey Month Four:

Limbo

SEPTEMBER 24, 2018

I am feeling a bit strange in my body, like there are now two sides of misunderstanding in me. One side doesn't quite understand what I want to be/how to read myself and the other side doesn't quite understand what others believe me to be/how to read me.

Maybe part of this process is not knowing where I'm going but knowing I couldn't be where I was before. I get ma'am-ed, girl-ed, and lady-ed by strangers and familiar people alike, and I'm truly not sure what the contextual clues are to inform these readings. I have short hair, no boobs, and wear masculine clothing. There is something that we subconsciously read about gender, and it's difficult to tell whether people say ma'am so as not to offend me (by calling me sir), or because there is only that subconscious reading. I think of myself as boy, but not man and not woman. I use she but not ma'am or lady. I am aware this is confusing for others to navigate, but I think it's important to self-critique how we address people respectfully and in a non-overtly gendered way until we know their gender.

Pronouns aren't necessarily permanent and it's important to be aware that certain gender changes happen at different paces. Well-meaning queer people/allies often assume (without asking) that the pronoun they/them is the default for any androgynous or masculine-leaning person. Being masculine or even identifying as a boy doesn't bring with it an automatic pronoun change. I still use she/her and have found people usually assume I have shifted my pronouns to they/them after surgery. Assuming or continuing to use they/them pronouns after clarification is still misgendering. We should always ask.

I recognize this is not everyone's experience, and that's totally okay. People should discuss gender pronoun preferences and identities with those around them. However, as someone who now experiences misgendering constantly after having a public gender change, I want people to be aware that changing one part of gender identity doesn't inherently mean changing the rest of it. I'm still figuring out how to be a she-boy and not a lady ma'am woman man. And how I'll feel if in a month I am drawn toward a different pronoun. But while I figure that out for myself, please practice or at least notice the gendered way you might treat people, whether you think you can read their gender or not.

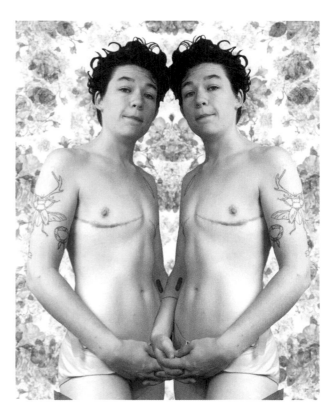

Afterword

Learning Never Ends

Gender, and all its millions of intersections, is incredibly charged: emotionally, personally, and politically. It's a topic that hits the most sensitive nerves in some and the angriest nerves in others. It ostracizes people from their biological families and creates loving communities of chosen families. It is a death sentence for some and a lifesaver for others. It gives power to some and makes others feel powerless.

The process of learning about gender is never finished. Our cultural understanding of gender is always evolving, and the genders of those around us (as well as our own) are always shifting.

It's okay to mess up and say the wrong things along the way—when you first experience someone around you changing their pronouns or name, you won't get it right every time in the beginning. It's okay as long as you're honestly trying (like, for real). You'll probably get better at adjusting with each person you know who changes their pronoun or name. You'll become more comfortable with someone you know who turns out to be gay.

Language changes over time, so the language used by your generation might now be outdated or even offensive (*transvestite* or *homosexuals*). Ask or research what the current, more appropriate terms are and don't defend what is now offensive. Language changes! When you think you've figured it all out, you haven't. Someone will always have something to teach you, intentionally or not.

We all come from different backgrounds, have grown up with different cultural understandings of the world, have different educations, are exposed to different types of people, and come to explore topics at different ages. It can be easy to forget that we learn in different ways and have different interests. **Ignorance doesn't always mean bigotry, but an unwillingness to learn is not okay.**

It can be hard to talk about these issues without being immediately politically divisive or alienating to those who don't have these conversations in daily life. We don't need to point out every infraction, call out every misstep, or shame anyone who hasn't been exposed to conversations about gender—that's not always an effective method of inviting connectivity or empathy.

However.

Sometimes anger is necessary.

Sometimes disengaging is necessary.

Sometimes we need to allow and ask others to have hard or triggering conversations on our behalf with those with whom we cannot. Not everyone has the patience or privilege to safely have these conversations, so those of us who can, should. If we are able (which sometimes we really aren't), we can ask in a loving and kind way to be open to hearing the experiences of others. Do not force someone to teach you about their experience if they do not want to offer it.

In writing this book, it's been a difficult balance to be gentle while not permitting disrespectful, harmful, and oppressive behavior. I personally don't think gentleness is always the right approach. You cannot fight hatred with gentleness, but I would hope if you're reading this book, you're not coming from a place of hate. However, I do believe it's important to **allow people the space to mess up while they grow**, and to simultaneously hold one another accountable when we're screwing up. Accountability is often uncomfortable, but so is change. Shaming those who speak incorrectly rather than engaging in conversation or recommending resources can breed silence, defensiveness, and a resistance to hearing a new perspective. I am very shame-prone. I have felt alienated plenty of times within my own community of radical queer people for being less versed in history or lingo, simply not knowing, or disagreeing. I shrink away easily when I screw up, and it's been an intensely difficult emotional process to try to be okay with misstepping or being accidentally offensive—it feels terrible. But it's a work in progress and if we can all get a little more comfortable being the ones who both say and hear "Hey, that wasn't cool," we might access more moments of learning than we expect.

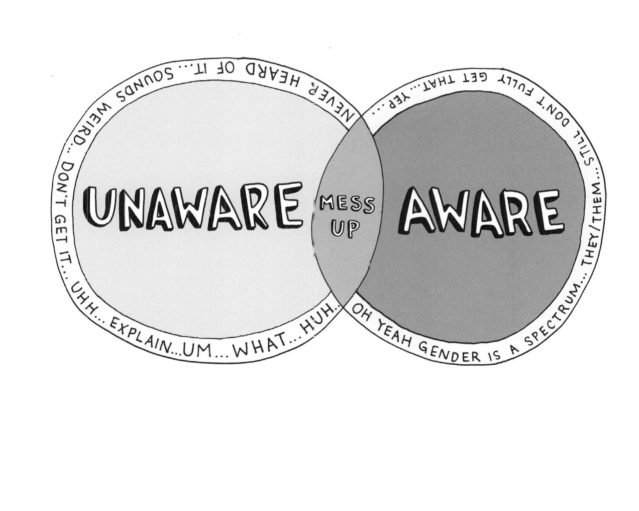

Resources to Expand Your Understanding of Gender

Books and Papers

Pick up any book by bell hooks and you're bound to find wisdom, insight, and intersectional perspective; this is a brief list:

- *Ain't I a Woman: Black Women and Feminism*
- *All About Love: New Visions*
- *Feminist Theory: From Margin to Center*
- *Talking Back: Thinking Feminist, Thinking Black*
- *The Will to Change: Men, Masculinity, and Love*

Assata by Assata Shakur

Bad Feminist by Roxane Gay

Bastard Out of Carolina: A Novel by Dorothy Allison

Between the World and Me by Ta-Nehisi Coates

Black Feminist Thought: Knowledge, Consciousness, and the Politics of Empowerment by Patricia Hill Collins

"Demarginalizing the Intersection of Race and Sex: A Black Feminist Critique of Antidiscrimination Doctrine, Feminist Theory, and Antiracist Politics" by Kimberlé Crenshaw

Fun Home by Alison Bechdel

Gender Outlaw: On Men, Women, and the Rest of Us by Kate Bornstein

Redefining Realness: My Path to Womanhood, Identity, Love & So Much More by Janet Mock

Sex Workers Unite: A History of the Movement from Stonewall to Slutwalk by Melinda Chateauvert

Stone Butch Blues: A Novel by Leslie Feinberg

The Body Keeps the Score: Brain, Mind, and Body in the Healing of Trauma by Bessel van der Kolk, MD

This Bridge Called My Back: Writings by Radical Women of Color edited by Cherríe Moraga and Gloria Anzaldúa

Women, Race, and Class by Angela Y. Davis

Online Resources and Hotlines

Everyday Feminism

everydayfeminism.com

Everyday Feminism is an educational platform for personal and social liberation. Their mission is to help people dismantle everyday violence, discrimination, and marginalization through applied intersectional feminism and to create a world where self-determination and loving communities are social norms through compassionate activism.

Asexuality Visibility and Education Network (AVEN)

asexuality.org

The Asexual Visibility and Education Network (AVEN) was founded in 2001 with two distinct goals: creating public acceptance and discussion of asexuality and facilitating the growth of an asexual community. Since that time they have grown to host the world's largest asexual community, serving as an informational resource for people who are asexual and questioning, their friends and families, academic researchers, and the press.

The Trevor Project

thetrevorproject.org

Lifeline: 866-488-7386 (24/7)

Text: text the word *trevor* to 1-202-304-1200 (4 to 8 p.m. EST)

Online Chat: *thetrevorproject.org* (3 to 9 p.m. EST)

The Trevor Project is the leading national organization providing crisis intervention and suicide prevention services to lesbian, gay, bisexual, transgender, queer and questioning (LGBTQ+) young people under twenty-five.

National Center for Transgender Equality

transequality.org

The National Center for Transgender Equality (NCTE) is a national social justice organization devoted to ending discrimination and violence against transgender people through education and advocacy on national issues of importance to transgender people.

The Silvia Rivera Law Project (SRLP)

srlp.org

The Silvia Rivera Law Project is a collective organization founded on the understanding that gender self-determination is inextricably intertwined with racial, social, and economic justice. They seek to increase the political voice and visibility of low-income people and people of color who are transgender, intersex, or gender non-conforming. SRLP works to improve access to respectful and affirming social, health, and legal services for the LGBTQ+ community. They believe that in order to create meaningful political participation and leadership, everyone must have access to basic means of survival and safety from violence.

National Resource Center on LGBT Aging

lgbtagingcenter.org

The National Resource Center on LGBT Aging is the country's first and only technical assistance resource center aimed at improving the quality of services and supports offered to lesbian, gay, bisexual, and/or transgender older adults.

Lambda Legal

lambdalegal.org

Lambda Legal is the oldest and largest national legal organization whose mission is to achieve full recognition of the civil rights of lesbians, gay men, bisexuals, transgender people, and everyone living with HIV through impact litigation, education, and public policy work.

Parents, Families, and Friends of Lesbians and Gays (PFLAG)

pflag.org

Uniting people who are lesbian, gay, bisexual, transgender, and queer (LGBTQ+) with families, friends, and allies, PFLAG is committed to advancing equality through its mission of support, education, and advocacy. PFLAG has 400 chapters across the United States.

interACT Advocates for Intersex Youth

interactadvocates.org

interACT uses innovative strategies to advocate for the legal and human rights of children born with intersex traits, including media work, strategic litigation, and the development of youth leadership. Issues of focus are informed consent, insurance, identity documents, school accommodation, discrimination, medical records retrieval, adoption, military service, medical privacy, refugee asylum, and wider international human rights.

National Center on Domestic Violence, Trauma & Mental Health

nationalcenterdvtraumamh.org

The National Center on Domestic Violence, Trauma & Mental Health provides training, support, and consultation to advocates, mental health and substance abuse providers, legal professionals, and policymakers as they work to improve agency and systems-level responses to survivors and their children.

Black Girl Dangerous

bgdblog.org

Black Girl Dangerous seeks to, in as many ways as possible, to amplify the voices, experiences, and expressions of queer and trans people of color.

Resources for Chest Binding

FtM Essentials: *ftmessentials.com/pages/ftme-free-youth-binder-program*

Point5 cc: *point5cc.com/chest-binder-donation*

Point of Pride: *pointofpride.org/chest-binder-donations*

These organizations offer free chest binders to qualifying individuals under age twenty-four who are unable to purchase a binder on their own due to financial circumstances.

Rebirth Garments

rebirthgarments.com

Rebirth Garments' mission is to create gender-non-conforming wearables and accessories for people on the full spectrum of gender, size, and ability. The line creates a community where all people can confidently express their individuality and identity. Their identity is that of QueerCrip, a politicized umbrella term that encompasses queer, gender-non-conforming identities, and visible and invisible disabilities/disorders—physical, mental, developmental, emotional, etc.

Rad Remedy

radremedy.org

Rad Remedy's mission is to connect trans, gender-non-conforming, intersex, and queer folks to accurate, safe, respectful, and comprehensive care in order to improve individual and community health.

Transgender Europe (TGEU)

tgeu.org

Transgender Europe envisions a Europe free from discrimination, where each person can live according to their gender identity and gender expression without interference and where trans people and their families are respected and valued. Transgender Europe is a membership-based organization. TGEU currently has 112 member organizations in forty-four different countries (as of March 2018).

Black Trans Advocacy

blacktrans.org

Black Trans Advocacy provides referral services, case management, and direct services within ten components served through their national advocacy network and state chapter coalitions: Community Outreach, Human Services, Education & Training, Health & Wellness, Economic Development, Community Outreach, Legal & Public Policy, and Faith & Healing. They also provide medical service grants.

Darcy Jeda Corbitt Foundation

darcycorbitt.org

The Darcy Jeda Corbitt Foundation provides transition assistance grants twice a year to transgender and queer individuals who want to legally change their name, start hormone replacement, or have gender-affirming surgery.

Association for Gay, Lesbian, Bisexual, and Transgender Issues in Counseling

algbtic.org/therapist-resource-listing.html

This is a list of therapists for LGBTQ+ individuals. The website also has an extensive resource list for mental health, legal, medical, and housing issues affecting LGBTQ+ populations.

FORGE

forge-forward.org

FORGE is a national transgender anti-violence organization that supports, educates, and advocates for the rights and lives of transgender individuals and SOFFAs (Significant Others, Friends, Family, and Allies).

Planned Parenthood

plannedparenthood.org

Phone: 1-800-230-PLAN

Planned Parenthood delivers vital reproductive health care, sex education, and information to millions of women, men, and young people worldwide. Planned Parenthood has over 650 health centers in the United States.

International Planned Parenthood Federation

ippf.org

IPPF works in 170 countries to provide health care related to sexual and reproductive health. Visit their website to locate an organization in your country.

National Eating Disorders Association (NEDA)

nationaleatingdisorders.org

Phone: 1-800-931-2237

The National Eating Disorders Association is the largest nonprofit organization dedicated to supporting individuals and families affected by eating disorders. NEDA supports individuals and families affected by eating disorders and serves as a catalyst for prevention, cures, and access to quality care. NEDA has free or low-cost support groups across the United States.

National Sexual Assault Hotline (confidential)

Phone: 1-800-656-HOPE

Online chat: hotline.rainn.org/online

RAINN created and operates the National Sexual Assault Hotline in partnership with more than one thousand local sexual assault service providers across the country.

Trans Lifeline

877-565-8860 (24/7)

GLBT National Hotline

1-888-843-4564

M–F 4 p.m. to 12 a.m. EST

GLBT Youth Hotline

1-800-246-7743

M–F 4 p.m. to 2 a.m. EST

GLBT Trans Teens Online Talk Group

glbthotline.org/transteens.html

Ages twelve to nineteen (Wednesdays 7 to 9 p.m. EST)

Fenway Health LGBTQIA+ Helplines

Ages twenty-five and older: 617-267-9001

Ages twenty-five and under: 617-267-2535

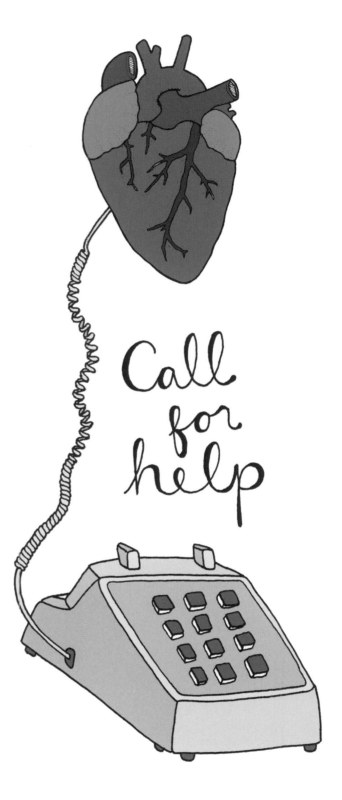

Call for help

Index

Acknowledgments

I'd like to primarily thank you, the reader. This book was made entirely from a desire to reach people in whatever moment they're in to feel connection or understanding, so thank you for reading it.

Thank you to Kate, Sarah, Sahara, and Solana for all their work on this project. To my friends who listened to my ideas and gave feedback.

To Elizabeth, Jay, Lucy, Claire, Aki, and Ashley, as well as the sensitivity readers and proofreaders for their help on this new edition.

To all those before me who made it possible to be writing so openly on this subject as a queer/trans person and to all those brave people who are continuing to fight for safety, rights, visibility, and equity for those who don't have their voices as easily heard. To my beautiful boys for inspiring me along this journey. To those who are genuinely trying to learn and work hard to understand others' experiences.

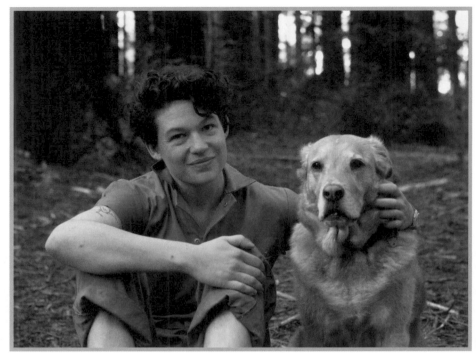

Chani Bockwinkel

Iris Gottlieb is an illustrator and author of *Seeing Science: An Illustrated Guide to the Wonders of the Universe* and *Natural Attraction: A Field Guide to Friends, Frenemies, and Other Symbiotic Animal Relationships.* She lives in Durham, North Carolina, with her dog, Bunny.

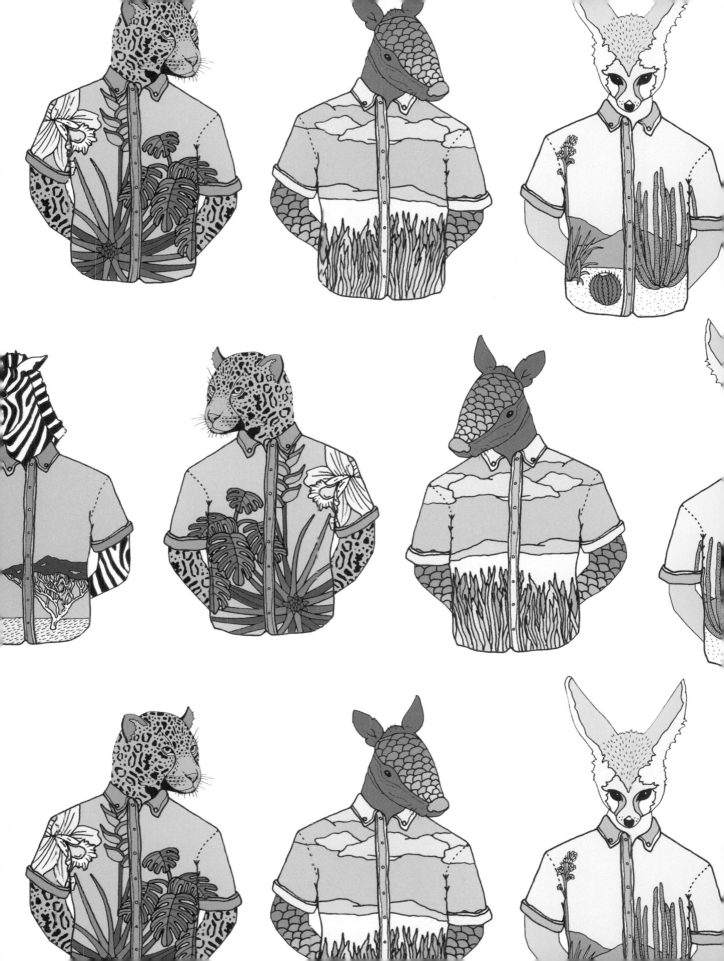

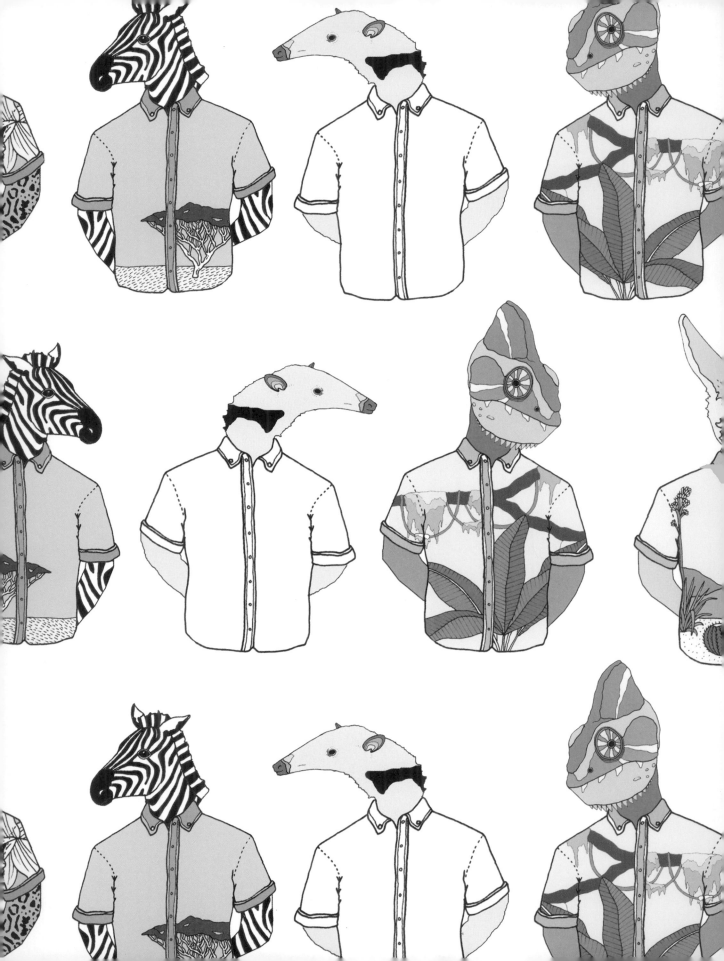

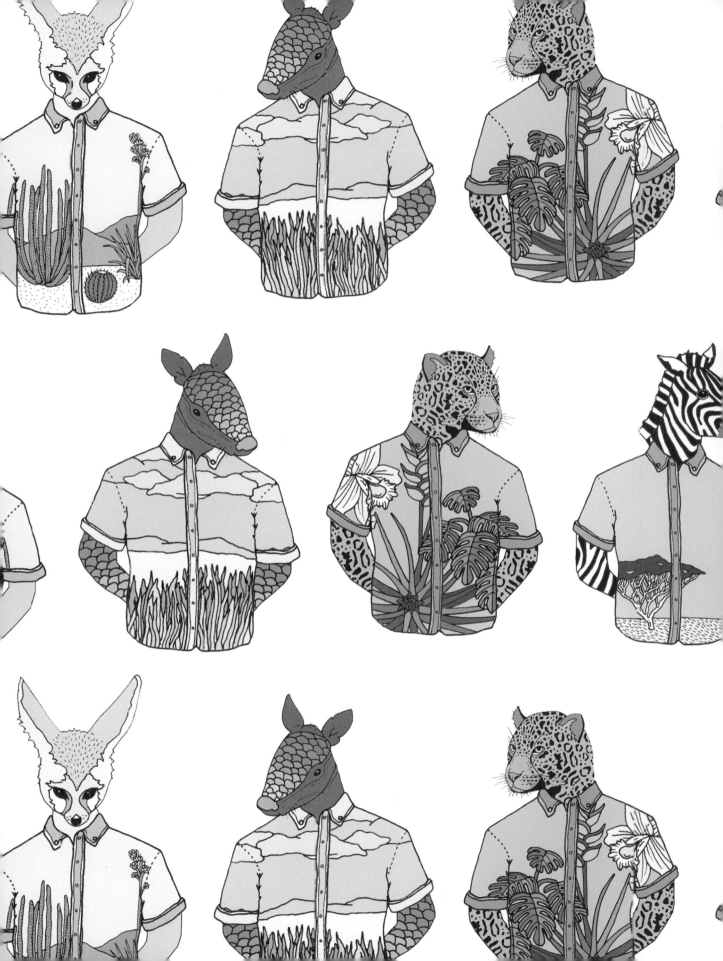